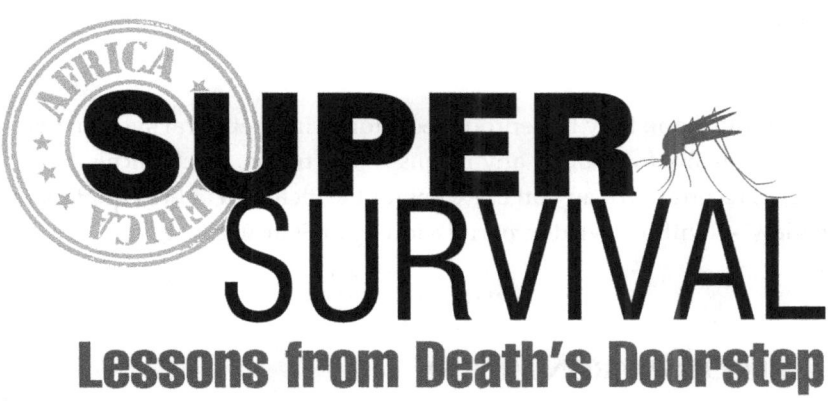

SUPER SURVIVAL
Lessons from Death's Doorstep

RON MEYERS

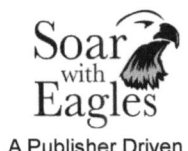

A Publisher Driven
by Vision and Purpose
www.soarhigher.com

Super-Survival:
Lessons from Death's Doorstep

Copyright © 2013 by Ron Meyers. All rights reserved.

ISBN-13: 978-0-9834528-6-7
Library of Congress Control Number 2013943682

No part of this book may be reproduced, stored in a retrieval system, or transmitted in any form or by any means — electronic, mechanical, photocopy, recording, or any other except for the inclusion of brief quotations in a review — without written permission from Soar with Eagles.

First Edition

OTHER BOOKS BY RON MEYERS
- *Habits of Highly Effective Christians*
- *Habits of Highly Effective Christians Study Guide*
- *Rise to Seek Him: The Joy of Effective Prayer*
- *Choose Your Character: 25 Bible Personalities Who Inspire Integrity*

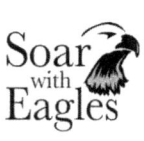

Published by
Soar with Eagles
2809 Laurel Crossing Circle, Rogers, AR 72758 USA
www.soarhigher.com

Design by Carrie Perrien Smith
Photography by Char Meyers
Editing by Millard Parrish and Carrie Perrien Smith

Printed in the United States of America

Contents

Acknowledgements v
More Than a Foreword vii
Introduction xiii
1. Israel: Initial Observations 1
2. Trio 7
3. Beauty 15
4. Words 21
5. Sedation 25
6. Bath 31
7. Support 37
8. Wounds 43
9. Lions 51
10. The Journey 57
Afterword 93
About the Author 97
Tools For Leaders 99
Other Books by Ron Meyers 101

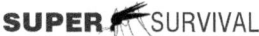

ACKNOWLEDGEMENTS

Char has again been a great blessing with her encouragement and I will always be grateful to our two sons who partnered together so that Dan could visit me in the hospital in Israel.

Millard Parrish was most helpful in the many times the manuscript went back and forth through cyberspace even before Carrie Perrien Smith put the finishing touches on it.

I am grateful to God for the privilege of sharing with the broader body of believers the lessons I learned through my sickness. May His name be forever praised.

I have worked with Soar with Eagles three times before. This time was no exception. I was coached and encouraged as my work was improved with editing. Carrie Perrien Smith has come through again with a publication that is artistically attractive and a fine piece of literature from a literary standpoint. I am especially thankful for the interesting way she used artwork on the front cover to hint about the contents of the book. Thank you Carrie.

Ron Meyers
Tiberius, Israel
July 2013

MORE THAN A FOREWORD

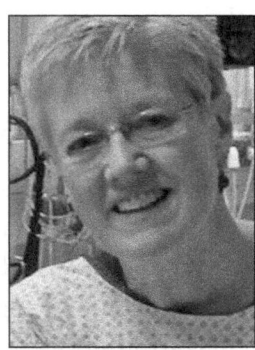

A message from Ron Meyers' wife, Char.

Near the end of October 2010, Ron and I had just arrived at an apartment in Tiberius, Israel. We intended to rest there between trips to Africa where we work. Immediately, we began preparing for a five-week trip to Rwanda for a nationwide series of Leadership Empowerment Conferences. We were already weary, but Ron progressively experienced a more severe headache and felt sore like he had the flu. Instead of getting better as our trip drew closer, he became increasingly ill. He would feel better during the day, but the nighttime chills and fever kept intensifying. This was the prelude to our adventure with malaria. We did not know it yet, but we were in for a wild and scary ride.

We were scheduled to fly to Rwanda late Sunday night. Late Friday night brought a frightening round of Ron being so chilled, then burning up with fever. I e-mailed a friend who was a family physician in Tulsa, Oklahoma. He replied, "It could be the flu. But it sounds like malaria to me."

Malaria

Though it was now 1:30 in the morning, I told Ron what the doctor said and insisted we go to the emergency room. This was the wee hours of Shabbat, the period of Sabbath from sundown to sundown. In Tiberius, the likelihood of finding a clinic or doctor anywhere but up on the hill in the Poriya Hospital was nonexistent. It was ten miles away.

I usually let Ron make these decisions, but it was now obvious he needed medical attention before we flew to Rwanda in less than forty-eight hours. To my relief, he agreed. "In the morning," he said. "Let's sleep now. Then we'll stop by the hospital before we go to the congregation meeting."

Ron is a good steward of God's financial resources and was concerned about the cost of the service. We had just made an expensive transition from South Africa. The next day (Sunday), we planned to head out of the country with our share of financial obligations. We did not want to use the cash we had budgeted for the trip.

Learning that it would cost about 300 NIS (Israeli shekels, roughly $80 U.S.) to be seen by a doctor, Ron hesitated. But I insisted that if we were going to Rwanda, we had to have medicine for him to get well as we faced a grueling schedule ahead. He finally agreed and was admitted for testing and treatment.

We had the immediate attention of the doctor and other staff. It was quickly confirmed that he did indeed have malaria. The doctor wanted to admit him into the hospital for twenty-four hours of observation. But again, Ron hesitated. He asked, "How much is this going to cost?"

Ignoring his question, the doctor persisted, asking if he had any rash. No, neither of us thought he did. Not to be deterred, she took hold of his trouser legs and jerked them up, one after another. I gasped, "Look at that!" Both ankles were peppered! At that, Ron realized it was important to yield to the doctor's expertise.

Ron will detail the events that followed. The escalation of difficulties came at us suddenly like a roaring storm. It was another major challenge that called for our best efforts in faith and prayer!

When we turn back and ponder all that happened, we are very

aware it was only God who had us in the right place at that time. It was only God who spared us Ron's death and the destruction of his teaching ministry. It is only God who brought us out on the other side strong enough to pick up again and move on to our assignments in Africa.

You can imagine the warfare against our spirits as we went through these events. Yet, in spite of these challenges, I look back and realize God was preparing me, speaking to me in several unique ways even before Ron went to the hospital. Those encouragements from God are what carried me through.

All I Needed Was an Onion

Friday morning, the day prior to our trip to the hospital, I headed out for my thirty-minute walk. I was already tired. And I was thinking about getting a few more groceries before that evening.

Shabbat is a significant celebration for the Israelis every weekend. It had become a highlight of the week for us. It begins on Friday evening with supper. Most businesses are closed on Saturdays, so traffic is heavy on Friday mornings as people do their last-minute shopping for the preparation of the Sabbath. Getting across

Char's Two Onions. These are the onions Char found on her walk on the day Ron was hospitalized. They were to her a sign of God's attention to detail and involvement in the difficulty in which they were engulfed.

town and in and out of grocery stores on Friday is never quick or easy. I groaned at the thought of having to do more shopping.

We had been invited to two different meals, one that evening and the other the following noon after worship. As I walked down the road, I moaned in my spirit, asking the Lord to give me grace. I lamented that maybe we should not have accepted the invitations when we were so busy.

Then I saw something in the middle of the road that hadn't been there just a few minutes earlier when I was walking the opposite direction.

Two onions! Really nice, solid and fresh, and not badly battered from having fallen in the street. I looked around. Certainly someone would be coming back to retrieve them. But there was no one anywhere nearby. What was I to do? I picked them up. With one in each hand, I fairly skipped all the way home. Continuing to think through my menus, I realized all I actually needed was an onion — one onion! God had provided more than enough!

Ron's warfare against death continued into Sunday, the second day. I carried the second onion to the hospital and set it on his bedside table. It said to me, "God is mindful; God is with us." He had provided the onions I needed without the extra burden of fighting traffic in and out of the stores. Surely He could take care of any other need; we just needed to trust Him.

Lessons

Ron and I have experienced some pretty difficult and long, drawn-out trials. The lessons we learned were always to be patient, to wait on the Lord, and to let Him do the fighting for us over a period of time. As Ron has written in this book, and earlier in *Habits of Highly Effective Christians*, it is important that we learn lessons from our experiences and let those lessons shape our lives for the future.

However, never had we been in such sudden and intensely terrifying circumstances as we faced now. Still, what we learned from those previous lessons continued to sustain us through these dark, turbulent hours. Little did we know, though, the significant lessons that we were about to learn through this ordeal.

I am married to a wonderful, godly man. He never lets a good lesson go to waste. And his commitment to apply the lessons to our life together has enabled us to become stronger over all our years of married life.

As Ron came out of his medically induced coma four days later, God began to show him lesson after lesson. He received a series of revelations during the recovery from the ravishing of the enemy in his body. They make up the heart of this book. He originally brought all these lessons together and outlined the chapters in his thoughts while he still lay flat on his bed in the intensive care unit. He knew these lessons were too good not to share.

As you read about our experiences and brushes with the searing attack of a vicious enemy and the gracious protection and enlightenment of a loving God, may the Holy Spirit encourage you as you face your next life-battle.

Char Meyers

INTRODUCTION

In 2006, my wife, Char, and I decided to commit the last years of our lives to training Christian leaders in the cities of Africa. We resigned our positions, sold our home and cars in Tulsa, and began a wonderful journey throughout Africa, traveling and conducting Empower Africa Christian Leadership Conferences. Over the years since then, we have met and worked with some of the most wonderful people, often in larger cities and at other times in smaller cities in remote regions throughout the continent.

Travel into the interior regions is difficult and dangerous to one's health — especially with rampant malaria and other diseases throughout Africa. In order to relate better with the people, we intentionally stay in the homes of our hosts, rather than in hotels. We also use local means of transportation. This contact with the people is an extremely rewarding learning opportunity. God has given us amazing friends in many countries.

> "Travel into the interior regions is difficult and dangerous to one's health — especially with rampant malaria and other diseases throughout Africa."

However, this lifestyle takes quite a toll on our bodies, indeed every part of our being. Normally after a series of seminars over a month or two, we have retreated to a rented apartment in Pretoria,

South Africa for a time of rest, refreshing, and regrouping. These times are absolutely necessary for our continuation in this work.

Recently, however, we have received invitations to conduct conferences in India and other parts of Asia. People in Europe are also contacting us. This drove our decision to begin taking rest and recovery times between work trips in Israel instead of Pretoria. This location allows us to travel with equal ease to Africa, Asia, or Europe.

In September 2010, we began our first such retreat in the town of Tiberius in Israel. It is a lovely town on the shores of the Kinneret, known to many as the Sea of Galilee. While working to prepare for this and future visits, we were also recovering from the recent and difficult strains of traveling in sub-Saharan Africa. And, at the same time, we were preparing ourselves for our next series of conferences scheduled for Rwanda in November and December.

Most tourists vacationing in Israel do not spend twelve days in a hospital fighting for their lives. That would not have been my choice either. But an excellent hospital very near Tiberius is where miracles took place, bringing me back from numerous life-threatening illnesses.

It is a high privilege to be enriched by difficulties, assess one's life and value system at a deep level, and then remain alive to act on what was learned. Each of the following chapters is my attempt to share some of the unique lessons that became clear to me through this most difficult, yet wonderful, experience.

These lessons may not be new to you, but they may provide an opportunity to review some valuable old lessons and deepen their impressions. It will be well worth recording my personal experience if you can gain insight into these lessons and benefit without going through such pain yourself. This is my personal story and some of the lessons I learned, or re-learned, through the crucible that almost killed me.

Char and I are so grateful for the medical team and attendants God used to spare my life and restore my health. As you look through Chapter 10: The Journey, you will see a collection of photos taken with many of these key people.

You can also see a series of x-rays that demonstrate the progression of the infection in my lungs, and then its regression. You will see the hand of God and the skill of a great medical team that turned the tide and snatched me from an early death.

Finally, many concerned and praying friends all over the world journeyed with me during these twelve days. It is sobering now to realize that people were fasting and praying for my recovery even as I struggled to stay alive hour by hour. Their communications with Char and our son Dan (who came from Canada to be with us) are also key factors in this story. I feel a great deal of gratitude for each one of them. Some of the notes they sent are especially uplifting. They are also included in Chapter 10.

For a few days, life for me could have gone either way. I could have died of malaria and resultant complications at age sixty-six. Indeed just a week prior to my experience, a twenty-nine-year-old lady, who had also contracted malaria, returned to Israel and died.

Why did God spare me?

Hopefully, the following pages will partially answer that question.

1
ISRAEL: INITIAL OBSERVATIONS

Years ago, before modern Israelis drained mosquito-infested swamps, Israel had a problem with malaria. Today, they still know how to effectively treat it. Israel is not, however, where I contracted malaria. It is where I was healed.

Ever since visiting Israel and particularly Tiberius in 2006, Char and I have especially liked the Galilee area.

Tiberius is a small city on the west side of the Kinneret (the Sea of Galilee). It is sometimes called simply "the lake." It is a tourist attraction in the northern part of Israel. The pace there is slower than the busy and highly religious Jerusalem or the racy, spicy, and modern Tel Aviv. One attraction is Tiberius' hot spring that continues to attract some of the Israeli and foreign tourists.

The trip on Highway 77 offers the first glimpse of the Kinneret as travelers cross over the crest of the hill at Poriya Junction. From there, the entire valley is visible, including the mountains on the east side. The scene is breathtaking. About three-quarters of the way down the hill, travelers reach sea level. The road leads to the lake, which is 209 meters (685 feet) below sea level.

The Romans selected this location centuries ago as a center for military activities and the administration of their colonies in the Middle East. Today near the Tiberius city-center, the large rocks used in Roman fortifications, buildings, and city walls still stand. They add a kind of romantic mystique to the city.

Jesus based much of His ministry in the northern part of Israel, especially in the Galilee area. This makes the Sea of Galilee an attractive holy site for Christians from all over the world to visit. Nigeria, for example, has a policy of helping their citizens make trips to holy sites abroad. Many Nigerians choose to travel to Mecca, but an average of 23,000 visit Israel each year.

In September and October 2010, Char and I were enjoying a rest period in Israel between our ministry assignments in Africa. We had completed a most exhausting assignment in the two Congo Republics followed by some time in South Africa. We were preparing for our next series of conferences in Rwanda in November and December.

We spent about six weeks in Tiberius preparing our vacation apartment for future use and regrouping. It was now the end of October. We were scheduled to fly all night on October 31 to Rwanda for our next series of leadership conferences.

However, I had recently become plagued by headaches that would not stop. My muscles ached. I experienced real discomfort for four days. Usually I am able to shake off a cold or the flu in about three days, but not this time. For several nights in a row, I experienced extreme cold chills and could not get warm. I was wearing warm winter pajamas under blankets and hugging a hot water bottle. Char even got in bed with me just to help me generate heat. I later broke out into a high fever, sweating profusely. That fourth day of feeling particularly ill (Friday, October 29), I realized I had something more serious that was causing severe and lingering symptoms. We decided it was time to get medical attention.

During the night, Char wrote to a friend of ours in Tulsa, Oklahoma who was a medical doctor. He concurred with Char's hunch that I had malaria. I was skeptical. I had regularly taken Larium, a malaria preventative or protector from contracting the disease. It had worked well for both Char and me during the previous four years we had been conducting leadership conferences in sub-Sahara Africa.

After leaving a malaria-infested area, we normally continue to take Larium as prescribed for several more weeks. Larium prevents malaria and also kills the newly hatching eggs that can produce another generation of the bacteria. Continuing to take the medicine prevents further malaria by dealing with the next generation before it matures. Contrary to our usual practice, however, we had stopped taking the Larium this time just after we departed from the Congos.

> "I thought I would get needed medicine and stay with the Rwanda schedule. However, to my disappointment, I was moved from the emergency unit to the hospital proper. Little did we know that the struggle for life was just beginning. I would remain in that hospital for twelve traumatic, difficult, and wonderful days."

The next morning (Saturday, October 30) marked the fifth day of solid headaches and body pain. It was the day before we were scheduled to travel to Rwanda. Char and I stopped at the emergency unit of the Baruch Padeh Medical Center in Poriya. The hospital was located at the top of the hill above Tiberius to the south and west. Poriya could almost be considered a suburb of Tiberius.

We were on our way to worship that Shabbat (the Sabbath or Saturday). I thought I would get needed medicine and stay with the Rwanda schedule. However, to my disappointment, I was moved from the emergency unit to the hospital proper. Little did we know that the struggle for life was just beginning. I would remain in that hospital for twelve traumatic, difficult, and wonderful days. Before it was over, I would be moved from the internal medicine unit to the intensive cardiac care unit, intensive care unit, and then back to the internal medicine unit for the last three days in the hospital.

I cannot boast about or acclaim the staff at the Poriya hospital enough. They are skilled, professional, competent, and business-like. And beyond that, they are extremely caring and helpful. Judging from their attitude and demeanor, they did not perform their duties begrudgingly or with a mere sense of obligation. Rather, these hospital staff members put their hearts into their work.

The staff is made up of a wide variety of ethnic and religious backgrounds. There are Jews, Moslems, and Christians from Europe, North America, Russia, Africa, and Israel — all are part of the colorful social mosaic. In the hallways, hospital rooms, and patients' dining rooms, I saw Jewish people, each with their own *kippah* or *yarmulke* (a small, round cap placed on the top of the head). I also saw Arabs with their traditional garb, flowing white robes and distinct headwear. I saw others dressed as one would see in any western nation today. In the hospital, everyone worked together in apparent harmony.

We had already noticed similar harmony in the city of Tiberius (a largely Jewish community) and also in nearby Nazareth (a largely Arab and partly Christian city). The various ethnic and religious cultures seem to live and mingle quite peaceably in both of these northern Israeli cities. In the hospital, I witnessed that they also work together happily and cooperatively as well. And patients are all treated equally well, regardless of ethnicity, religion, or economic condition.

What I had read in the world press was so different from the reality I found and experienced! I came away from my twelve-day adventure at Baruch Padeh Medical Center in Poriya with the sense that Israel should receive better treatment in the world's propaganda wars. It is sad the press doesn't tell of the real Israeli life that I observed each day in the intensive care unit. If they would, the people of the world would have a far more accurate and positive impression of Israel's lifestyle, living standard, work ethic, and peaceful happiness together.

I am not a journalist; I am a teacher. But if I were a news writer, I would take up this theme in my reporting. I hope I can make it clear that Char and I both are quite favorably impressed with what we have seen of the people and lifestyle of Israel.

Learning about Israel firsthand from a hospital bed forced me to examine the unfairness of judging a place and a people without direct personal contact. We cannot trust the world press for accurate representation of a nation and its people. The press emphasizes negative information to make dramatic newscasting. It's too bad that positive news is considered mundane.

But, as I have seen it, it is possible for people of different ethnic and religious backgrounds to live together in harmony. These are a few of my thoughts as I contemplate the difference between the Israel I saw in the hospital and the Israel one sees or reads about in the world media.

What I learned about Israel during this experience is only one of the many lessons learned over those twelve days. There were also other major lessons God helped me understand during my struggle.

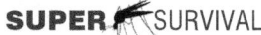

2
TRIO

People who know me well know that I am task and goal oriented. I am motivated by purpose as I try to accomplish what I understand to be God's plans for my life. Accordingly, I am impatient when something interferes with fulfilling these objectives. I had planned to be in Rwanda. Whatever interrupted those plans had to be overcome as soon as possible.

Instead, through the three stages of my illness, the trio — diagnosis, treatment, and recovery — God was prepared to teach me some valuable lessons.

Upon entering the emergency room, I was led to a bed behind a curtain. Char sat down beside the bed, and the lab technician took his first vials of blood for the normal procedure of testing. The emergency room was not overly busy. The physician on duty that morning, Irena Ovichka, a lady of Russian background, arrived within minutes. She listened to our explanation of exposure to malaria in the Congos and ordered a number of blood tests.

Shortly after the doctor left, the technician came in again. He was a vivid example of manual dexterity. I watched with utter fascination as he quickly filled nine little vials with blood from a vein in my arm. I have never seen a medical technician draw blood, insert the next tube, and repeat the process so quickly. The little tubes were flying from his fingers to the tray on the bed with the skill of a juggler. He soon gathered his second collection of vials and left. Thankfully, this fascinating entertainment helped me endure my wait.

The doctor returned about an hour later announcing that I may indeed have malaria. She arranged for me to be admitted to the hospital's internal medicine unit while I waited still longer. Knowing this would take some time, Char went on to the congregation meeting and shared with our new friends what was happening. While she was gone, I changed into the hospital pajamas and waited. Eventually the malaria diagnosis was confirmed, and they began treating me.

I was eager to begin treatment. I needed to prepare for our departure to Rwanda. I wanted to get the problem fixed quickly! The malaria had already been doing its deadly damage for just over three months. I did not want to wait another day before giving a strong medical counter-attack.

Yet, like any decision in life, good diagnoses that lead to good decisions are better than fast decisions. Getting a proper diagnosis requires waiting and testing. Treatment is best when treatment is correct.

As in the medical arena, every problem we face in life is best handled after proper diagnosis. If we seek first to have an accurate understanding of the difficulty, its treatment will require less effort with more effectiveness and better results.

The second part of this trio, the treatment for malaria was not a bad experience. It consisted of taking two white pills every eight hours. That evening, the congregation pastor and his wife came by. I was able to sit up and chat with them. I was responding to treatment well enough that I assumed I could probably be released the next day. All I needed, so I wrongly assumed, was to get this medicine in me quickly so I could move on to my important responsibilities in Rwanda.

But that was not the case. Throughout the next day, my strength and, even more seriously, the ability to breathe declined steadily. I was gasping for each breath by evening. What was happening to me?

This disease had been working silently in my body for ninety-six days. It had done more damage to my health than we suspected. The malaria was quickly and, until now, undetectably destroying my tissue, attacking and infecting my organs. While being treated for malaria, a secondary yet uglier problem was raising its head. It seems I needed to learn some additional long-suffering.

Treatment for malaria was fairly simple. But treatment for a very serious long-term disease was another matter. It needed further diagnosis. However, they began treating me immediately to deal with the breathing problems while preparing me for more diagnostic tests.

> "I was gasping for breath before they put the mask on me. The mask made it even more difficult to breathe. I wanted to cooperate, but horror gripped me with a desperation I had never experienced before."

Three events stand out to me regarding the treatment I began receiving. One was an attempt by the nurses to cover my face with a rigid mask that did not allow any air inside except what the mechanism controlled. I was gasping for breath before they put the mask on me. The mask made it even more difficult to breathe. I wanted to cooperate, but horror gripped me with a desperation I had never experienced before.

Next was the trip to the intensive cardiac care unit. There, I received the strongest sedative I have ever experienced. The morphine knocked me out and enabled them to take more x-rays. They revealed the gravity of the problem in my lungs. I had serious pneumonia in both lungs, which led to a life-threatening disease called Acute Respiratory Disease Syndrome (ARDS).

The third was having a ventilator in my throat. This was bittersweet.

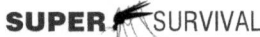

It was terribly uncomfortable, yet it saved my life. The same ventilator that irritated my throat also delivered oxygen and air to my dying lungs. After three days on the ventilator, it was removed. Thankfully, I was sedated for forty-six hours of these three days.

The diagnoses for both the malaria and the respiratory diseases had been made correctly. The treatment was accurate and effective, though not pleasant. I was learning more about the value of patiently going through the steps necessary to make a correct diagnosis and also undergo proper treatment. And now, I was to learn about the third member of the trio.

My primary physician in the intensive care unit eventually announced that the malaria and pneumonia had been defeated and my lungs were being restored. He also said, "And tomorrow you will begin recovery."

What? If I was well, could I not get out of the hospital right away?

I was again disappointed at a delay. I had anticipated that when the treatment was over, I would be free. Not so. Not by a long way. I failed to understand the third necessary phase of the restoration of health — recovery.

From my experience with malaria and the other life-threatening illnesses, I am trying to review a life-lesson about waiting for the right time; more properly, it is a lesson on allowing time. I find that I must relearn this lesson from time to time: allow time for each stage of what I am doing. Since this experience, I am trying to apply this principle appropriately to other areas of my life.

I am a man of action. I want to do what needs to be done to solve a problem as quickly as possible. Waiting for an accurate diagnosis was a struggle for me, but it was a necessary phase. I am much more comfortable with the treatment phase — taking action — even if this means enduring some discomfort and taking time. I would prefer not to take much time on treatment, but I tolerate it better than the process of diagnosis. Now I had to learn to wait some more as I entered the recovery period.

Whatever difficulty, problem, or challenge we are working through, we need to establish new habits and patiently recover. We need to plan for a recovery period and be patient with the process, just as much as we need to allow time for diagnosis and treatment.

In my case, after I got over the initial disappointment of knowing there would be days spent in physical therapy (PT), I realized the wisdom of the physician's statement: tomorrow I would begin the needed recovery.

Physical therapy focused on two main objectives:

- Strengthening my breathing capacity in order to expel all residue from the double pneumonia.
- Strengthening my body so I could walk again.

My first minutes of daily physical therapy, therefore, focused on getting my lungs and diaphragm functioning normally. The therapist pounded on my rib cage from all sides to loosen the deadly excess in my lungs. I learned four exercises to increase my breathing capacity and strengthen my diaphragm. Over the first several days, a large amount of accumulation was gradually eliminated from my lungs.

Later each morning, I worked on learning to walk again. It took two nurses to assist me that first morning as I painstakingly worked my way down to the foot of the bed, lowered myself from the bed, and then sat in a chair that was waiting for me. It took about six minutes to get to the chair the first time. The next day, however, I did the same thing in about one minute.

I sat up in the chair for approximately five hours that first day after the ventilator was removed. Just sitting up seemed like a wonderful dream come true. I felt as if I had become a big boy and was doing something wonderful.

I am amazed at how much like a little boy I had become. Every activity centered totally on me. Every accomplishment, great or small, was a great triumph, and I felt everyone should know about

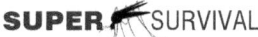

it. It was a good lesson on child psychology and should make me more sensitive to the feelings of children.

That second day after six hours of sitting up in a chair, I also hung onto the foot of the bed and stood up almost unassisted for my bath. I thought it would be good preparation for starting to walk the next day. All I did was hang on and remain more or less upright. As I collapsed into bed at the end of the project, I was ever so proud of myself. I wanted to tell the world, "I stood up on my own!"

All together, three physical therapists helped me. The third physical therapist was the most helpful because she pushed me the hardest. She worked with me for three days. We exercised lungs and diaphragm together. And when we went for walks in the hallway, she pushed me to go farther.

Because of my own self-motivation, few people need to push me; I sufficiently push myself. I usually require more of myself so that I can more than satisfy others' expectations or desires. Not so, however, with this powerful little lady therapist named Ofer. You can see a photo of the two of us in Chapter 10 that was taken as we went down a hall during one of my "walks."

The most defining moment during my therapy with her happened when we, accidentally I thought, entered a stairwell. To my surprise, she did not back out of the stairway saying something like, "Oops, that is not a hallway; it is a stairway." She instead entered and told me to climb up a flight of steps. In my bravery and courage, I complied. I began the ascent in my manly way. I stepped up a step and brought my second foot up to that step, hesitated, and then took another courageous step up.

Instead of boasting about my wonderful accomplishment, she said something like, "You said you were a marathoner. I want you to move that lower leg and foot past the other one onto the higher step and go up these steps in the normal way."

I hesitated, grinned at the challenge, and climbed the flight of about fifteen steps. I held lightly onto the handrail, not to pull myself up, but to steady myself and make certain that I would not fall. I was quite weak. When I finished the descent, I was thoroughly proud of myself.

I have often taught my students that we weaken people by being too easy on them. Now I was on the other end of that instruction. I still believe that is good advice.

My physical therapy continued under my own supervision after release from the hospital. Each day, I forced myself to walk periodically around our vacation apartment a little bit. I made my own bed, brushed my own teeth, shaved my own beard, and took a shower using my own strength. I felt a bit like a little boy again — proud of each new and grand accomplishment.

I learned again that developing patience along with resolve and determination is greatly beneficial. It also can be an enjoyable challenge.

The entire trio I've described in this chapter — diagnosis, treatment, and recovery — applies not only to medical situations, but also in many other life and work-related challenges. Each problem we face requires:

- Careful research to assist in making good decisions — the diagnosis of the problem
- Correct action — treatment — which is sometimes painful but only possible after doing the first stage correctly
- Careful and patient recovery, hopefully without setbacks.

What project are you up to now in life? Are you learning to follow an accurate process to arrive at an accurate diagnosis when making decisions? Are you willing to go through the treatment stage of carefully applying the needed remedies? Then toward the end of your project, do you leave space for yourself to recover?

Each stage in this trio requires patience. I think of this as the ability to anticipate certain desired expectations while being content with

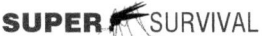

the delayed gratification and fulfillment of those expectations. I learned that I tend to focus on the treatment or correction stage and am impatient with the diagnosis and recovery stages. I hope to become wiser because of this experience.

I mentioned in the introduction that you may not learn anything new in this book. Rather, you could expect a practical review of important lessons. These lessons are not new or even that profound, but they are extremely important. Give yourself time to make a good plan for recovery. Then change, improve, grow, or do whatever is needed to implement the plan for success beyond the initial correction. We may stumble or even fall at times in life. But with God's help, we can boast, "Wow, did you see that great recovery?"

3
BEAUTY

Usually a man of my age has matured to the point that he is not so dependant on people speaking gently, carefully, or in a tender way. Generally, we expect an older person to have outgrown exaggerated concern about his own feelings.

But in my sickness, I became more sensitive to the way people treated me. Wrestling with the physical weakness and pain, plus the emotions that go along with being seriously ill, I found myself preoccupied with my own feelings. I became the little boy I referred to earlier.

I came to appreciate so much the tender display of love and care shown to me throughout this whole experience as a patient. In my greatly weakened condition, I realized that the kind character and gentleness caregivers express toward their patients is vital to the success of the healing process.

Reflecting on this, it occurred to me that an inward character of competence, warmth, and professionalism is much more important than outward physical beauty. I fortunately never encountered any incompetent nurses or other personnel during my hospital stay. But as I thought about this very important principle, I concluded that I would rather have a plain-looking, competent, and courteous nurse than an outwardly beautiful, incompetent, and impatient one.

True beauty is inward. It is the beauty of character and competence rather than mere external appearance. What we are on the inside and how we treat people — in other words, our character — is much more important than how we look on the outside.

Our appearance is indeed a partial reflection of the kind of people we are. To a degree, it is important that our appearance be as good as conveniently possible without extreme preoccupation with mere peripheral matters such as clothes, hair, and personal hygiene. However, character development is more important than appearance. It is even more vital to success than the shallow emphasis people often place on mere outward show.

Happily, I experienced and noted this higher standard of beauty in the attitudes, actions, and professional demeanor of my healthcare givers. I attribute much of my healing to this type of beauty displayed toward me, and I want to learn from their example.

An especially poignant manifestation of this beauty occurred in one of the most vulnerable positions a man can be in.

> "I recall the nurse who assisted me to the bathroom for the first time after days of no movement in my bowels. Even though exposed in a way that otherwise would have totally humiliated me, I surprisingly felt comfortable with the process. Her professionalism, kindness, and sensitivity to my helpless situation impressed me."

I recall the nurse who assisted me to the bathroom for the first time after days of no movement in my bowels. Even though exposed in a way that otherwise would have totally humiliated me, I surprisingly felt comfortable with the process. Her professionalism, kindness, and sensitivity to my helpless situation impressed me.

Because of these qualities, I regard her as one of the many beautiful persons who attended me while in the Poriya Hospital.

As I reflected on the principle of inward beauty, I remembered a friend of mine who majored in music at university. One of the early classes he took was music appreciation. I never realized how important it is to appreciate things until my friend described that class to me. Students learned to evaluate the tempo, harmony, variety, and accuracy of attack on each part of the melody. By the end of the course, these students knew the difference between good and poor music. It taught them to appreciate good music; they would no longer be satisfied with poor music.

Similarly, we should study the behavior of others. Our purpose is not to judge them; that would be wrong. Rather we should observe others to learn the behavior and attitudes we consider to be beautiful. Then we can apply such lessons to our own lives. While developing inner beauty ourselves, we can reject the selfish and inwardly turned attitudes that we do not appreciate.

As I evaluate myself, I still find too much unpleasant character within that I would like to change. I would much rather reflect the beauty of personal maturity and the ability to think of others.

While I lay in my bed observing the beautiful behavior of our caregivers, I reminisced on my past experience in teaching ethics. I like to define the study of ethics as the study of morally beautiful attitudes and behavior. Here the same principle — beauty in motive and action more than in appearance — is made clear.

I taught ethics several semesters in Korea. In the beginning of that course, we discussed the fact that an act or behavior can be either beautiful or ugly, depending on the factors behind the behavior. A behavior can be either pleasing or displeasing to the observer at first glance. However, the intent of the behavior, the risk to the actor, and the benefit or loss to those being affected should all be part of the evaluation. A person's motives must be factored in to appreciate the beauty of good attitude and behavior.

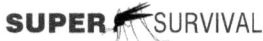

Compare these two examples of similar behavior. One young man might risk his life and jump toward a weak, hobbling woman walking in the street and knock her down in the process of pushing her away from an approaching car that could have killed her. Another young man with evil intent might jump toward a weak, hobbling woman walking in the street in order to knock her down under the approaching vehicle. Both of these young men jump toward and knock down hobbling old women. However, would you say that their behaviors were equally pleasant or unpleasant? No.

Who would claim that both men had the same ethical system? One risked his life to save the old woman; and the other selfishly, even cruelly, tried to kill her. This starkly demonstrates the contrast between beautiful and ugly conduct that necessarily goes beyond the appearance — knocking down old women — and addresses the motives which make the behavior attractive or unattractive, saving or killing.

There in the hospital, I compared that perspective on ethics and the care our nurses and doctors gave their patients to the way we each treat others during day-to-day interaction. Only once did I ever see a nurse act unkindly toward a patient. It was an extreme example, and it is easy to understand that the nurse may have been irritated. I mention it here only because it is such a sharp contrast with the good ethics, kindness, and gentleness I found throughout my experience in the hospital. Pondering this event also prompted a subsequent change in my own reaction to this same difficult situation.

A mentally imbalanced and very troubled patient across from me in the intensive care unit continuously called out and cried loudly. This happened all day long and for several nights all night long. I had earplugs so I could more or less endure the noise, but the caretakers did not have that advantage. Hour after hour, she continued her irrational behavior with a very loud and abrasive voice.

One early morning, a nurse came on duty after the rest of us had endured this inconvenience for many hours throughout the night. After hearing her cry out two or three times, the newly arrived nurse turned toward the patient's bed and mocked her, unkindly repeating what she had cried out in an equally plaintive voice. This was the only time I saw unkindness — ugliness, not beauty — during all my time in the hospital.

During the time the deranged patient was causing such a stir, I asked how people like that could financially afford such good care in the hospital. I was informed that Israel has socialized medicine, so everyone, rich or poor, receives the same treatment. As one night dragged by, I pondered the fact that I, a foreigner, was paying for my hospital expense while this young person disturbed so many and interrupted my sleep. Yet she received the same loving and gentle care with no expense to her. Was this fair?

While I was complaining inwardly about this, I decided I should duplicate the kindness the Israelis showed to this weaker member of their society instead of complaining about the inconvenience to me. Even outside the hospital, I had noticed a fair number of older and handicapped Israeli people on the streets of Tiberius. They rode their electric wheelchairs or walked slowly using a walker and enjoyed the same pleasant scenery the rest of us did.

So in the middle of the night, I recognized that I needed to learn to appreciate the ability of Israel's strong citizens to help the weak ones I observed all around me. What I saw on the boardwalk in Tiberius by the Sea of Galilee and then in the hospital room was the same beauty revealed in behavior. Even in my weakened condition, I decided I would value and appreciate true beauty — what I was seeing.

I then pondered this question: What do I need to do differently to attain such a patient attitude, beautiful behavior, and kind demeanor? The beautiful attitude of the caretakers compelled me to re-evaluate the importance of character development during those twelve days in the hospital. But what self-control, patience, kindness, gentleness, concern, and helpfulness did I need to cultivate? Even with God's help, how would I do that? What changes did I need to make so that as I travel through the rest of

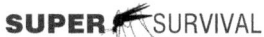

my life, my behavior encourages the development of the good in others around me?

I continue to search for the answers to these questions. The mere fact that I rediscovered the need to be more patient with the weak is hopefully another milestone for me. I will continue to seek to appreciate and pursue the more important type of beauty. This is another valuable lesson of life learned near death.

4
WORDS

When I was a little boy, I became offended when people said unkind things to me or about me. This is the normal human reaction to unkindness. My mother knew that as life went on for me, she could not control what people around me would say. She taught me a common saying that helped me then: "Sticks and stones may break my bones, but words can never hurt me." She wanted me to develop thick skin. Instead of letting people's words hurt me, I could just brush off the teasing or taunting. I understood then and still understand her point today.

But as life has progressed, I have decided that words do hurt us. Actually, they hurt a more important part of us than the physical part. They injure more deeply.

This chapter is therefore a further treatment of the theme addressed in the previous chapter on beauty. The emphasis on our words here, however, is made separately from that chapter. Words are behavior — a special category of behavior. And they can be particularly beautiful or ugly; uplifting or discouraging. Physical behavior can be observed and interpreted, but words are a more intentional form of communication, whether in affirmation or spoken in unkindness.

I survived malaria in November 2010. In just ten months of recovery, my body was strong again. Now almost three years after dismissal from the hospital, I still run and exercise with free weights regularly. Thanks to God's intervention and medical science, many human

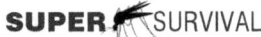

illnesses can be healed or cured. Bodily injuries heal so naturally that without thinking about it, we are well in a matter of weeks. A sprained ankle heals in several weeks. Even a broken bone can heal in just six weeks. Furthermore, a bodily injury usually is visible and elicits sympathy or concern from others.

Bodily injuries are more easily understood than emotional scars that lie beneath the surface. The victims do not always understand emotional injuries. But with careful treatment, a kind friend can draw out those pains and help to heal the inner person. Without a doubt, emotional hurts can be more devastating than broken bones.

My application of this principle leads me to say that we each need to exercise self-control so we don't hurt people. What I mean by self-control is the ability to control our tongues. We need to refrain from saying something terribly destructive — something that cannot be recovered, erased, or redeemed without resolving the damage of the harsh words.

We need to control our words so that we do not hurt others. A lot could be said about how to cope with or handle the unkind words people say to us. But the thoughts I was pondering in the hospital revolved around determining how to protect those we love from our own hurtful words.

The incident that triggered these thoughts occurred about 8:00 a.m. one morning. I was far enough into my recovery to be sufficiently alert to appreciate what was happening around me. I am the curious type. If I am in a dentist's chair, I ask for a hand mirror so I can watch the action. If I am being given a medical exam or a physical test such as an echocardiogram, I am always trying to see the screen. I want to watch. I want to learn.

To help pass the long nights, I watched the screen from time to time displaying my vital signs on a panel beside my bed. I even requested they turn the screen slightly in my direction so that I too could watch it with the nurses when they stood at the foot of my bed. I could see my temperature, heart rate, blood pressure, pace of my breathing, percentage of oxygen in my blood, and the activity of my heart. I was happy and even a bit entertained by making my own personal observations. The whole process was quite intriguing.

A new team of professionals arrived at 8:00 a.m. each day. As I stated in the previous chapter, one of them spoke unkindly one morning to a distressed young female patient. Meanwhile in my part of the ICU, the first thing that same unkind person did was to deliberately turn the screen. Now only those at the foot of the bed could see it; I could not. So I asked, "If you wouldn't mind, would you be willing to turn the screen just a little bit so I can watch it too?" I understood when the nurse said, "The screen is for us to watch …" But then the nurse added the unkind, cutting, and unnecessary: "… not for you!" I knew the screen was for them, but did I need to be told it was not for me?

> I was reminded of an even more hurtful incident that had occurred in my life years ago. What bothers me the most about that earlier incident is that it was I, not the other party, who said the unkind and regrettable words.

As the hours passed, I pondered that brief conversation. I tried to evaluate my own feelings that resulted from what the nurse said to me. It changed me. I wanted to make sure I was never guilty again of doing the same thing. I did not want to make another person feel like this nurse had just made me feel. Unfortunately, while reviewing the situation, I was reminded of an even more hurtful incident that had occurred in my life years ago. What bothers me the most about that earlier incident is that it was I, not the other party, who said the unkind and regrettable words.

I lived abroad at the time. A leader at the headquarters for my organization asked me to relay a message to a local colleague about a policy. I was the foreigner, and the colleague was a national.

The colleague did not like the message and began to argue with me. Into that already-volatile conversation I needlessly, unkindly, and regrettably inserted these words: "I do not believe this is a matter for our discussion; rather it is an announcement of a decision."

There are many complex and complicated reasons why my cross-cultural relationship with that colleague was difficult. The lines in the chain of command were not clear, and it created an authority problem. The relationship was already thorny without my poor choice of words that morning. But adding those words to the conversation was counterproductive, unkind, and unnecessary. I wish now I had not said them. I also realize these words sprang from unresolved frustration I harbored toward my colleague.

Even now, I am in an awkward position with a neighbor I did not choose but whom God has allowed into my life. We have different opinions about some issues involving our adjacent apartments. I have thus far succeeded in not expressing my disappointment. I do not want to argue with this person so I must hold my tongue. I must also resolve to live with an unpleasant situation without becoming resentful.

So as I review the life lessons learned during the fight for my life against malaria and its ensuing diseases, I will add this one about carefully choosing our words. Life is short. Cooperation and harmony are pleasant. Competition and wrangling are not. My experience in the hospital has reinforced my determination to choose my words carefully and consider how my words might make the other person feel. I could ruin things by saying something unkind, and I would rather not do that.

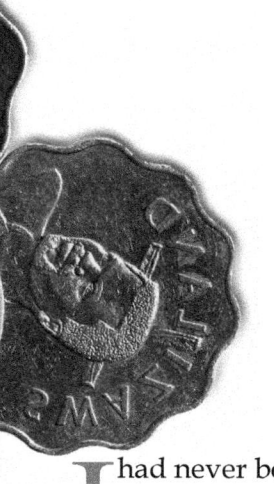

5
SEDATION

I had never been sedated for such a long time as I was from the evening of November 1 until the evening of November 3 (a total of about forty-six hours). This long medically induced coma was necessary to keep my esophagus from reacting to the intrusive ventilator inserted in my throat. The esophagus is designed to immediately reject any foreign substance. In order to stop the normal reflex, I was kept under sedation.

Coming out from sedation — becoming conscious once again — I experienced something else I never had before. I went from the perfect bliss of ignorance to awareness of problems in and around me. I began thinking again, even thinking seriously about this process as it was happening.

Sometime during the early hours of semi-consciousness with the ventilator system in my mouth and going down my throat, I became aware of my discomfort. It seemed to be exacerbated by two problems. It felt like a wire designed to hold the apparatus together in my mouth was catching on my gums below my front lower teeth. And it seemed as though a thread that was part of the mechanism was dangling down into my esophagus. The whole apparatus was tickling my throat and esophagus, causing me a good deal of discomfort.

I tried to bring my situation to the attention of my caregivers. It was difficult because I had no voice and I was weak. My caretakers evidently thought that I didn't like the device in my mouth and throat (which is true, I did not). However, I was totally unable to communicate the more serious difficulties: the wire cutting my gums and the thread tickling the unseen depths of my esophagus.

The tickling and irritating wire and thread sensations continued. Nature finally took its course. While lying on my back in total weakness and vulnerability, I vomited into my own mouth and the beard that had grown since arriving at the hospital. My face was covered with vomit. I feared I was about to breathe vomit down into my lungs and would drown in it. Too weak to sit up and unable to speak, I struggled but only weakly. Finally I had to breathe. So with no other alternative, I gulped into my sensitive respiratory system.

Wow! Wait! What is this? Breath after breath of oxygenated sweet air! And no vomit!

I had feared I was about to suck vomit from my mouth and face down my throat into my lungs, but I was wrong. I had failed to understand or trust the ability of the ventilator tubes to deliver clean air from outside the narrow confines of my vomit-filled world.

Now, months after taking time to reflect, I realize that what I perceived then to be a thread hanging down my esophagus and a wire cutting into my gums was a misperception. Neither thing existed. It was simply the discomfort of the ventilator I felt as I came back to reality. But we live at the level of our perceptions. As I lay there with my mouth full of vomit, it was very frightening to think — to perceive — I was about to breathe it down into my lungs.

I can learn from this. I can learn to question my own perceptions. I can learn to trust my caregivers. Even more importantly, I can learn to trust God. He is able to deliver the breath of life to our drowning souls as well as to our pneumonia-filled lungs.

What was the difference between the peaceful hours that had just passed and the present tickling, inconvenience, and "near drowning" I was experiencing?

I was becoming aware of my world. Now I was waking up after

having been sedated. My senses had been intentionally dulled, and now that dullness was wearing off. My nervous system was beginning to function normally. Sedation is not normal; I was leaving the abnormal sedated state and again becoming aware of physical realities.

Would I have rather reverted back to the comfort of sedation? Part of me said yes, and part of me said no.

> "I feared I was about to breathe vomit down into my lungs and would drown in it. Too weak to sit up and unable to speak, I struggled but only weakly. Finally I had to breathe. So with no other alternative, I gulped into my sensitive respiratory system."

Here is the heart of the issue. The fully conscious state is normal. When sedated, we are in an abnormal state. We are out of touch with reality, usually by a conscious choice. We take the sedative and lose awareness of our own environment and the real world. It is intentional.

In the hospital, sedation is a necessary therapeutic reprieve. But in the world of daily living, there is another kind of sedation. It results from an immature frame of mind. This more abstract type of sedation is an escape from responsibility. It makes us comfortable, relieving us from having to be sensitive to the needs of others around us or of being useful to anyone.

To be spiritually or morally sedated is to become like the proverbial ostrich and to put our heads in the sand. By doing this, we ignore the needs around us, intentionally choosing to be passive and unaware of the needs. By taking no action, we become sedated — out-of-touch — with reality.

The normal, mature adult who is a fully functioning personality desires to be helpful to others. The mature person is not content to be totally preoccupied with personal matters; he wants to be useful. So the fully functioning personality will take the action necessary to emerge from sedation. He will inform himself so he is aware of what is happening around him.

Medical treatment may include sedation, but what causes moral or spiritual sedation? What causes a person to be unaware of the hurts, pains, and sorrows that make up the reality around us?

I thought of these three "sedatives" as I considered the difference between the comfort of sedation and the awareness of personal responsibility experienced during consciousness. The following is by no means an exhaustive list. You will be able to identify more than just these.

The first is *ignorance*. Not to be informed, not to make ourselves aware, or not to educate ourselves is one form of sedation. If I do not care about what is happening around me, I do not listen or read. I simply remain preoccupied exclusively with living my own life. I can become comfortable in my ignorance. Such sedation is happiness; ignorance is bliss. But does such a life have worth?

A university colleague of mine used to laugh on his way out of his office near mine as he moved toward his next class, "Well, let's go stamp out ignorance." He did not want his students to be sedated by ignorance. He wanted them to become useful. For anyone in this information age to be ignorant of the needs of people around him is to be like an ostrich with its head in the sand.

In actuality, at the approach of trouble, ostriches lie low and press their long necks to the ground attempting to become less visible. Their plumage often blends with sandy soil. From a distance, it can give the appearance of burying its head in the sand. The illustration of the hiding ostrich is even more relevant when we liken it to ignorance. It is foolish to not be aware of danger. Hiding and refusing to be aware does not decrease the danger or make us useful to others.

Apathy is the second sedative. Apathy is to know but not to care. This kind of sedative is even less kind than ignorance. We know of the suffering, pain, or sorrow around us. However, we choose to ignore it or are emotionally unprepared to consider our need to respond.

Ignoring something we know is different from being ignorant of it. Nevertheless, apathy may sedate us with essentially the same result as ignorance — we do nothing to relieve suffering, pain, or sorrow. With ignorance, we make no effort to know and are comfortable not to know. But with apathy, we know but choose to ignore. Both are selfish, but apathy is more so. Both avoid the responsibility of the strong to help the weak. Both hinder the growth of character that belongs to the caring.

I also thought of a third sedative: *selfishness* — a preoccupation with or concentration on self. Such a person knows the needs around him or her but remains focused on his or her own personal comforts, desires, and concerns. The selfish person does nothing to alleviate the suffering, pain, and sorrow around him or her because those needs compete with his or her own interests. Selfishness is a refusal to recognize responsibility for others.

Compare apathy to selfishness. Apathy is usually a less intentional form of not caring, whereas selfishness is more intentional. Apathy is almost an emotional inability to care rather than an intentional choice not to care. Apathy can also include an inability to care about one's own needs. It can prevent a person from helping others while causing them to assume that others will and should help the people in need.

Being sedated and then gradually becoming aware of the reality around me made me realize how apathy sedates us. We become insensitive to the reality around us and refuse to accept our responsibilities.

The sedative which sedates each of us differs from person to person. And the degree to which we each are sedated varies from time to time, even within each individual. For each of us, it will be a different mix. We must each learn to identify the sedative that is most likely to keep us from being useful. And then we must refuse the sedative.

It is necessary to decide that usefulness to others around us is of greater value than our own personal comfort in our sedated state. We may also decide to become responsible for ourselves and others. If we are to mature and influence the real world around us, we must avoid or escape from any sedative that separates us from needs around us. We discover the joy of usefulness when we seek to either remain in or reenter reality.

Obviously we cannot meet every need or alleviate all the suffering around us. We can, however, deliberately choose which needs to address and how we should respond to the others. Our response may just be a caring prayer. But we cannot afford to totally ignore these needs if we want to become sensitive and caring persons.

As I gradually became more and more aware of the reality from which I had been separated, the teacher in me emerged. I considered how I might share these ideas, hoping that my experiences and observations might also help others. After being "asleep" for the previous forty-six hours, I did not sleep at all that night — not one wink.

All night long, I pondered what had been happening to me. I thought about the convenience of sedation in contrast to the responsibilities entailed in consciousness. I also began to think of other lessons I had learned in addition to these reflections on sedation and consciousness.

This book was born in my mind that night. Throughout the sleepless hours, I "wrote" it. God and I conversed at length. This dialogue continued the next night when again I could not sleep. As a result of those two nights of contemplation, I soon wrote down the nine chapter titles and the main thoughts to be communicated in each chapter.

6
BATH

I had never had a bath in a hospital that I could recall. With some obvious mental discomfort, I wondered what would happen when the nurse got to the private part of my body. My mother, when I was a baby, and my wife are the only women who have ever touched me in that area of my body.

In a situation that was potentially very embarrassing, I appreciated the way my nurse approached her work. Sonluk, the nurse on the evening shift in the intensive care unit, bathed me a total of three times. When she came to the private part of my body, she simply proceeded with perfect professionalism and maturity, giving me no undue concern.

Later as I was talking with her, I reflected on the experience of the bath. I told her I had never been touched in that area of my body except by my mother and my wife. She nodded understandingly.

God enabled me to use this as an opportunity to tell her about the chastity Char and I both held to until we were married. This young lady was astonished that I had never had sex prior to marriage and let me know that she agreed with this value. We were able to take the conversation even a bit further which was very meaningful and both mature and polite. I came away from the conversation with the conviction that what we had discussed needed to be included here. I felt others would benefit from the things she and I talked about.

As an aside, but an important lesson nonetheless, it was not until a day or two later I learned that she was not only of a different ethnic group but also a different religion than I. This caused me to break a stereotype in my own mind. I learned again that each individual we meet should be evaluated on his or her merits, not only as a part of the wider group to which they belong. There were a remarkable number of similarities between our two value systems.

As a result of this conversation, I became even more thankful for the total freedom and trust that Char and I have in our relationship. People who believe and practice the teaching of the Bible have greater levels of trust, security, and satisfaction in the intimate part of their marriages than do non-believers.

This has been supported by statistical findings of researchers over the years. I also received the same outcome in 1986 from my own quantitative and statistical survey. Hollywood in the United States and Bollywood in India try to make their portrayals of sexual activity appear stimulating, exciting, and satisfying; but according to concrete statistics, believers enjoy a superior experience and greater overall satisfaction.

It was not just a coincidence that Char and I were both sexually pure when we got married. Each of us had the advantage of having godly parents who trained us in the teachings of the Bible. And each of us decided we wanted to be chaste until marriage. We wanted to offer our marriage partner an intentionally inexperienced sex partner so we could make our discoveries together. The plan worked wonderfully. We married in 1969 and have enjoyed many years of fidelity and maintained a trust of each other.

There were many times we each could have had sex before we were married. For example, Char had one experience in which she was alone with a young man in his car, parked by the side of a lonely road. They were being modestly affectionate. After some brief time, he placed his hand on her breast. She immediately stiffened and moved away suggesting it was now time to go home.

Her response was not decided in that moment of excitement, which would have been too late. Good decisions about sexual behavior are not made during the heat of passion. Rather her response was based on a firm resolve she had made earlier that she would refrain from sexual intimacy until she was married.

I had numerous similar opportunities that I declined. Once when I was the student pastor of a rural church during my senior year of Bible college, a young lady came to visit me. Her demeanor, politeness, and expressions indicated to me that she was making herself available for sex if I was interested. I was not.

Another time when I was the associate pastor of another church, a young lady came to my house to tell me how worried about me she had become. At one point in the conversation she placed her arms around me and said, "I am so concerned about you." Right away she was escorted politely to the door and was gone. Pastors especially — and it is good advice for everyone — should avoid being alone with a member of the opposite sex unless it is their spouse. If necessary, make sure to meet in a public environment.

> "It was not just a coincidence that Char and I were both sexually pure when we got married. Each of us had the advantage of having godly parents who trained us in the teachings of the Bible. And each of us decided we wanted to be chaste until marriage. We wanted to offer our marriage partner an intentionally inexperienced sex partner so we could make our discoveries together."

Neither my wife nor I have ever been sorry that we made decisions to remain pure and that we had executed that decision repeatedly.

Even after years of marital happiness, there are still numerous opportunities for sexual activity outside of marriage. One time in the lobby of a hotel in Antananarivo, Madagascar, a pretty young woman approached me and asked me if she could be my wife while I was there. I showed her a photo of Char and explained that I was already married to the most beautiful person in the world. I asked, "Do you think I would throw away our happiness just for a brief time with you?" I then turned and walked away. Another time in Eldoret, Kenya, a young woman made a similar offer and I gave a similar response.

Is it easier to exercise self-control now than before I was married? I don't think so. When I travel without my wife, I am alone for long stretches at a time. It requires a conscious effort to keep my mind focused on the reason for the trip. I occasionally think about how my life's work and my relationship with my wife and our sons would be ruined if I let down my guard.

Does it become easier to resist sexual temptation when you get older? I am sixty-nine years old (as of July 2013), and I thought by now it would be a non-issue. But I was wrong. I still have to exercise discipline to keep my mind on what is good, righteous, and noble. I don't want to be a dirty old man. I do not want to live only at the animal level. There are loftier and better things to do with our lives than become predators or even to yield to the temptations of others. No, it does not become easier. If anything, knowledge of the pleasures makes the temptation even stronger.

So what exactly are the benefits that belong to those who remain pure until and faithful after marriage? There are many, but I will mention three.

One is that neither Char nor I have ever worried or needed to worry about the faithfulness of our partner. Not only do we enjoy each other when we are together, there are also many hours during which we enjoy the memory of our last encounter and then the anticipation of our next one. During this time, we flirt, tease, and enjoy the feelings of pleasurable satisfaction before we come together again in sexual intimacy. Even so, the trust and lasting satisfaction of fidelity outweighs the joys of our intimate times together.

The second advantage is that during an encounter, we never have to think about any other encounters we or our partner may have had. She is mine exclusively, and I am hers totally and only. We would be extremely jealous if we thought someone else was sharing the pleasure we share just between the two of us. Even in our thoughts, we refuse to imagine what others do in the privacy of their own bedrooms. Char and I have reflected that we wish every couple could be as happy together as we are.

> "Does it become easier to resist sexual temptation when you get older? I am sixty-nine years old, and I thought by now it would be a non-issue. But I was wrong. I still have to exercise discipline to keep my mind on what is good, righteous, and noble."

The third advantage is that our commitment to chastity before and fidelity after marriage frees us from all concerns about sexually transmitted diseases. This may occur to me because of our travels in Africa. We meet many AIDS widows and orphans. We know of entire societies in which children are raising children because their parents all died of AIDS. I also ensure the use of brand new needles any time my blood is tested or inoculations are given. I am even careful where and how I get my hair cut so I will never have to worry about getting AIDS.

Why am I willing to speak and write so openly about this subject? The answer to this question lies in understanding the influence of role models. Think about the bad models who are willing to speak openly and spread their vulgar interpretations, especially in the media. Would it be wrong for some of us to testify of the advantages of doing it right?

It has always seemed unfortunate to me that Hollywood can be so open and forthright in portraying its interpretation of unhealthy and destructive sex. Yet because of modesty, Bible believers never talk about this subject. They lose the chance to proclaim the excellent wonder of the joys of love-making in marriage. The younger generation misses the positive influence we in the older generation could be for them.

What benefit is there for you in reading a chapter like this? I would like to think there are several. Chastity is something you can appreciate and celebrate, not only for application in your own life, but as a benefit to those around you that you may influence. Do you have children? Can you influence them at an early age to value chastity? Do you have nieces, nephews, friends, or neighbors that you could bless with information that would help preserve them from evil? Or, if it is too late to establish any goal for chastity, could or would you repent of the past and determine to remain chaste and faithful in the future?

Certainly chastity is worth celebrating and helping others to commemorate. Freedom from guilt and destruction is a value worth living and modeling for others. So is freedom to enjoy pleasing God and one's spouse.

Over the years, God has given us many friends who have blessed us with models of chastity, faithfulness, and fidelity. And He has given Char and me many opportunities to share these truths with others. Sharing life with others and encouraging one another in godly living are values and lifestyles to which God has called us. In this next chapter, you are about to read of those who truly supported us during our hour of severe trial in Tiberius.

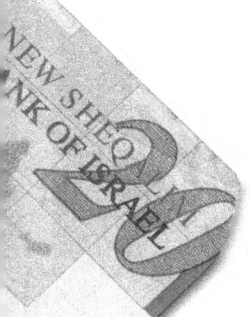

7
SUPPORT

Several weeks after I was released from the hospital, I consulted with the doctor regarding my new medications. I asked if the three medicines sedating my heart could be reduced. More than three weeks had passed. I was again doing routine exercises and lifting weights, and my muscles were becoming stronger again. But I could tell that my heart was not working like it had before. I moved in a sluggish way and did not have my former energy. The sedatives were too successful, I thought.

But the doctor was adamant; I was not to stop the medications!

Then, for the first time in my intense struggle and recovery over the past weeks, he explained what had happened the traumatic night of Monday, November 1. About an hour after I was put into a medically induced coma and the intrusive ventilator tubes were inserted in my throat, my body reacted further to all the trauma and medications.

My heart began to race at 200 beats per minute.

The atrium (upper chamber of my heart) was fibrillating, quivering instead of pumping, a condition I had lived with for six years. But, in addition, now the lower heart chamber (ventricle) was beating way too fast.

Ventricle tachycardia, a rapid ventricle beat, could lead to ventricle fibrillation. When both the atrium and the ventricle are quivering instead of pumping, death follows rather quickly.

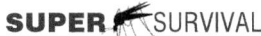

My six years of atrial fibrillation had already caused me concern. My heart had served me well through rheumatic fever as a five-year-old, hundreds of miles of training runs, and thirty marathons (two of which I ran after I developed atrial fibrillation). Now, in addition to atrial fibrillation, this was a new and more dangerous development.

In this follow-up consultation with the doctor, he said I was to continue the medicines that slowed my heart down. Hopefully this would keep me from experiencing ventricle tachycardia somewhere, sometime when I could not get the immediate attention I might need from cardiologists. Thankfully, help was available that night in the hospital; but what did the future hold?

For the first time in my ordeal, I came face to face with the severity of what I had come through and what I was now facing. This new heart condition was probably a permanent reality. I thought I had just come through the valley of the shadow of death and was rejoicing. Now I realized I needed to learn how to live with the fact that I am never very far from this valley.

My entire outlook, career plans, and goals in life needed to be adjusted in view of this more serious heart condition. I was facing a major paradigm shift. Various emotions began to bombard me. I wondered how this was going to affect my life's work. What I had just heard was more than a bit disturbing.

When I got back to our apartment, I shared this news with Char. She immediately saw I needed encouragement. Without flinching and in keeping with her loving ways, she began to help me prepare to move on in life with this new set of physical conditions. She began helping me think through the adjustments we would be facing together. She gave me just the support I needed at that moment.

Char has always been watchful and helpful without making me overly dependant on her. God intends that mates love and respect each other. To be supportive is part of that mix.

I was grateful Char affirmed and encouraged me through my valley and helped me adjust to what I thought would be my new reality. Char's support made my life more livable, enabling me to adjust and move forward. In the months that followed, my American cardiologist and family physician agreed with me that my medications could be reduced. To my personal satisfaction, this has allowed me to regain much of my former energy.

> "My entire outlook, career plans, and goals in life needed to be adjusted in view of this more serious heart condition. I was facing a major paradigm shift. Various emotions began to bombard me. I wondered how this was going to affect my life's work."

Char was by my side, encouraging me from the very beginning of our ordeal. It was she who had continued to insist I get medical attention even when I hesitated because of the expense. She was the one who helped me overcome part of my natural reluctance to see a physician and spend money on myself that we were trying to conserve for use in Rwanda. Her God-given wisdom and courage saved my life then!

Never have I appreciated Char or our two sons more than I do now. Under the pressure of making trips up the mountain to visit me twice each day, coping with life in a new foreign culture, and other unexpected responsibilities, Char refused to give me up. She contended in prayer, gathered prayer support both locally and around the world, and maintained her confidence that I would live and not die. Many were the hours she struggled alone.

When our sons Joel and Dan learned what Char and I were going through, they agreed that Dan should make a quick and unscheduled trip to Tiberius from Canada. He would represent both sons in giving Char and me some much-needed support. Although he could be with us for only a week, Dan was a great help and comfort to both of us. And Joel's frequent communications further added to the strength we received from our two guys.

> *In our leadership conferences, Char and I teach that if there is anyone in the world who wants you to succeed, it is your spouse. When spouses encourage each other, they can accomplish almost anything together.*

In our leadership conferences, Char and I teach that if there is anyone in the world who wants you to succeed, it is your spouse. I take this to be self-evident in any healthy marriage relationship. When spouses encourage each other, they can accomplish almost anything together.

It would not matter whether others encouraged, believed in, and heartened me; if Char did not, I would not be happy. Her smile of favor and cheering me on more than compensate for the normal disappointments, misunderstandings, and hurt feelings that arise in daily life in an imperfect world.

I have often thought I was the most blessed husband in the entire world. Now I am certain of it. I delight to support her, and she is happy to encourage me. These treasures make both of us very rich indeed.

What does a person do when his or her spouse is not supportive? I know of some dear people who somehow have learned to live without the emotional support of their spouses, but I do not know how they do it.

If you are not yet married, here is my appeal to you: base your search and prayers for a spouse on matters much more important and profound than only physical attraction.

Perhaps you are already married but either have lost or never have had a deeper emotional, intellectual, and spiritual connection with your spouse. Please consider developing it at any cost. There are many books and materials available to help us continually improve our marriage relationships.

If you are married and have a deep emotional connection with your spouse, maintain, guard, value, and protect it with tenacious fervency.

Our spouses know us better than anyone else does. If we will let them, they can be an enormous source of good advice and helpful information. They see things we do not see. They hear things we do not hear. Their critiques are valuable to us. But more to the theme of this chapter, our spouses can be a source of unconditional support and encouragement. You need that. Your spouse needs that.

I wish I could write or say something that would move the men and women of the world in the direction of enjoying what Char and I have experienced in our support of each other. It is possible. Mutual cooperation and affirmation between spouses can be cultivated. We can learn to *turn to* each other instead of *turning on* each other. I want that for you too.

So whether you are married or not, consider taking the steps appropriate for you to enjoy this very prized source of continual and unconditional help. Life is tough. Difficulties come our way. People misunderstand us. Disappointments happen. Learning to affirm your spouse and letting your spouse encourage you can be a great source of strength.

Not only was Char's, Joel's, and Dan's support invaluable. So too was the support we received from friends and the body of Christ near and far away. It contributed much to Char's courage and my recovery. Our new friends in the Tiberius area were a frequent blessing to both of us.

Char also got the word out by Internet through e-mail and Facebook. People all over the world were praying for us. As quickly as people

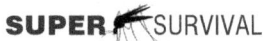

learned of our spiritual, emotional, and physical battles, they communicated back with Char in an almost endless stream of e-mails and Facebook posts. The support of prayer and flow of communications we received from family and friends throughout this crisis sustained us. It was invaluable in my recovery, and it strengthened Char's ability to survive the intense stress. She encountered the possibility of becoming a widow and, with the help of our friends, faced it down!

We highly value the way our friends upheld us. Because we consider them such an important part of our healing and survival, we want to share some of their expressions of love with you. Chapter 10 contains samples of the supportive e-mails and Facebook exchanges Char sent and received. I've included a sample of the e-mails I received after I was released from the hospital and shared with my friends the outline of *Super-Survival.* I share them with you so you can observe the power of encouragement, strength, and the help you too can give to someone in need.

Char has her own stories to tell about how God encouraged her through her trauma in the two intense weeks of my sickness. She has encouraged me so much in writing this story. Perhaps now it is my turn to encourage her to write her stories about her own adventures and experiences and the ways God spoke to her through Scripture.

Long live support for others!

8
WOUNDS

God loves us so much that He is willing to allow pain into our lives to improve us. Over the years, I have learned that He is more interested in our development than our comfort.

Throughout my entire experience in the hospital and since then, I never once have felt any conviction from either God or my own conscience that my illness was the result of any sin or wrongdoing on my part. Rather, I perceived this occurrence to be allowed by God as an opportunity for personal, moral, and spiritual refinement. God has used even this extremely difficult experience in my life — something bad and very painful — for a very good purpose.

During the toughest days in the hospital, I thought that if this was life, I did not want to live any longer. Yet, I've had an opportunity to reflect on the experience during these months after my release from the hospital. I acknowledge that this was part of His character-development plan for me. As a result of what God allowed, I could be and hopefully will be a better person. His wisdom is beyond me. His plan for character development is working. At least I certainly want it to work; otherwise I suffered for no reason.

We do not love suffering or like it even a little; but in many instances, we learn to appreciate and love the purpose or ideal for which we suffer. It seems that deep within the human psyche, God has built the potential for difficulties to test us and bring out the best in us. Our loving Father has created us with the potential to allow wounds to make us better.

I would not have chosen to contract malaria. I would not have chosen to allow it to incubate and ravage my organs for ninety-six days before I realized I needed to seek medical treatment. I would not have planned to inconvenience my wife and our sons with my sickness. I would not have chosen to suffer such extreme agony.

I certainly would not have spent many hours arranging a five-week conference schedule working on the Internet with six different hosts in Rwanda only to toss the plans in their entirety out the window. Nor would I have chosen to inconvenience these hosts and the people they had invited. I would not have chosen to do all this again, starting all over to reschedule and plan the Rwanda series of conferences.

Yet, I expect at some future time to be able to look back on the whole process — including my personal, spiritual, and character development through the malaria attack — and see how it was, as a whole, ultimately good. In order to understand this, we need to learn to distinguish apparent good from ultimate good.

Comfort often is apparently good. It seems good anyway. But suffering can be ultimately good because it is part of a larger process of refinement, development, and improvement. Wounds are intended to be ultimately good.

For those who trust the Lord with all their hearts, not leaning on their own understanding, and submitting to God in all their ways, He promises that He will make our paths straight. But if the favor of God and His blessings, protection, and care cause us to assume we deserve them, we have reached a wrong conclusion.

Why do we tend to think all should go well? Human beings are not promised that life events will always be easy. What if we lived in a world without wounds — a world that we might think of as perfect or superior? We would not learn to trust God like we can in the world that exists with the possibility of setbacks. The ease with which we would live would ruin us. We would not grow in character. We could become selfish and preoccupied with only our own happiness.

Praising God when things are going well glorifies Him and brings a level of happiness. But when things are not going well and we still give glory to God, the quality of our praise to Him pleases Him indeed.

God is not content to let us continue in our present level of maturity. From His point of view, we are each still a work in progress. As any creator or craftsman, God wants each of His productions to become masterpieces. Our character development is His handiwork.

The developmental process works especially well when we submit to the training. Our heavenly Father is very near, extremely interested, and intimately involved. He disciplines those He loves. He compliments us when He allows difficulties. He has higher ambitions for our refinement than we do for ourselves. His wounds are faithful.

We can depend on God to be actively involved in every situation into which we invite Him. Furthermore, since He *is* good, we can expect Him to be working *for* the good in every circumstance. The Apostle Paul says it this way: "In all things God works for the good" (Romans 8:28). Verse 29 goes on to say that the good that God is producing in us — to conform us to the likeness of Christ — is a very worthy goal. God can take even an apparently bad situation and work for ultimate good in it so perfectly that we might think the situation itself was good.

I don't believe that apparently bad situations are good, but I believe they can produce ultimate good. Bad situations do develop. Just because God successfully works for an ultimately good result in those apparently bad circumstances, it does not mean the situation itself was good.

We suffer sometimes from our own mistakes or the unkindness of others. I would not say either that God *created* those bad situations, though He did create a universe in which those situations could develop. Yet I delight to say that, in whatever situation I might find myself, I can count on God to work in it for ultimate good.

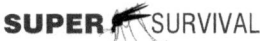

When we see beautiful character develop through suffering, we may want to ask "Why don't we suffer more?" rather than "Why do we suffer?" I am not a sadist or masochist wanting to heap more suffering on myself. Rather, along with you, I am struggling to understand and appreciate God's ultimately good purpose in allowing good people to experience bad events.

I cannot explain why suffering draws us closer to God and causes us to love Him more. But suffering can have this result. Malaria had this result in me; and I learned it is best to yield to the process.

> **I felt like God was very close, holding, cuddling, or hugging me very closely.**

I have no way to explain what I am about to say, but this is what I felt during many of the hours of my sickness. I felt like God was very close, holding, cuddling, or hugging me very closely. I never felt His presence depart. And even now when I recall the experience, I also recall that unexplainable sense of God's closeness and love.

The process of being wounded and comforted qualifies us to help an increased number of people. Each time we suffer, we increase our ability to influence others. The trials we experience qualify us to comfort those with similar experiences. In other words, our hardships greatly increase the number of situations in which we can empathize and speak with understanding to hurting people. I have met people who have never suffered, and I find them shallow for this very reason.

There is another outcome of my encounter with malaria as well. I am now able to speak to any other malaria victims or survivors with an increased degree of understanding. I understand how they feel, can demonstrate more genuine sympathy for them, and know how to help them in and through their suffering. These abilities all are additional qualifications for life and ministry I gained as a result of my victory.

You may recall the situation I shared in Chapter 4 in which I became more sensitive to being hurt by other's words. I learned in my sickness that when emotionally low, you may become more susceptible than usual to being hurt by words. Recalling those hurtful feelings motivated me recently to apologize to someone who was ill whom I unintentionally hurt with a remark I made.

So I confess that I still accidentally say unkind things that hurt others. I have a long way to go, but failures are not a reason to stop trying to use kinder words. Even with my setbacks, I still hope my experience of suffering will continue to lead me to be more sympathetic in this regard. If I were not trying to be careful with my words, I would probably hurt even more people than I do.

Suffering could make us bitter, hard, and angry with God and everyone else around us. But we can choose otherwise. We can choose character development and other ultimately good results of our suffering. All it requires is an attitude of accepting and submitting to suffering. This is ultimately much better than rejecting the suffering and the lessons God wants to teach us and the changes He wants to make in our lives.

Look at the results of injuries and setbacks in the lives of those around you who have learned to submit to them and have tried to learn from them. We like what we see in the patience, sensitivity, and care such people display even though we would not choose the process through which they developed these beautiful qualities.

The work Char and I do takes us to nation after nation of Africa. We have also traveled and ministered in Europe and Asia. We have seen uncomplaining, faithful, intelligent, and sincere people patiently face insurmountable difficulties and win. One of our hostesses in the Democratic Republic of the Congo had malaria. Another of our hosts in Uganda had a son, a college student, suffering with malaria. People suffer. But if we are isolated from situations like these, we are not aware and therefore not as sensitive.

Though we learn more from what we experience than we do from what we observe, we still can learn much from the things we

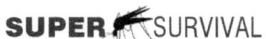

observe if we try. Westerners do not encounter firsthand the suffering that most of today's human population experiences as part of the normal process of life. Travelers have the advantage of seeing and learning from their experiences if we try.

God uses the apparent bad in this world, though not created — yet allowed — by Him, to turn us to Him for relief, learning, and improvement in character. The all-wise, all-powerful, and all-loving God is able to take either punishment for sin or common reversals of life in our world and turn them into ultimate good.

In my sickness, I acknowledged that the world we live in — a world with its malaria, parasites, germs, and bacteria that infest our bodies and destroy our health — is superior to a world without those difficulties that God could have created. Look at the good that has come to the human race as a result of facing and winning life's challenges.

God is the sovereign Lord. He does in the universe what He wants to do. The world as it exists is the result of flawlessly wise and careful planning. He intentionally planned an environment where mankind could and did exercise free will. When that results in evil consequences, man must be responsible.

God never does anything inconsistent with these three qualities: wisdom, power, and love. So I must logically conclude that what exists is best. If that were not the case, He would have lovingly, powerfully, and wisely created another kind of universe where what now exists would not exist.

What exists at this stage in God's ongoing plan is the best of possible worlds for now. If it could have been better, a perfectly wise, loving, and powerful God would have made it better. God is smarter than we are. He knows what is best. The end result in mankind's character development will be superior to what would have existed in a universe created without the potential for evil. We can see God uses it for good. King Jesus will eventually make things much better. That too is a part of God's eternal plan.

Why must man work by the sweat of his brow? Hardships and toil of our daily work can remind us of the harmful consequences of wrongdoing or lack of growth. They help us develop qualities like perseverance and diligence — qualities we would not have if everything were soft and comfortable for us.

Why did God increase pain in childbirth to women as a result of Adam and Eve's sin? Why must it be so stressful to bring a lovely child into the world? If our response to God is correct, the intensity of the pain a mother endures can be used by Him to strengthen the love she has for her newborn. It can also remind us of Adam and Eve's failure that introduced sweat and suffering. God graciously gives us the occasional reminder to live circumspectly before Him.

Why are soldiers who suffer loneliness, fatigue, and hardships among the most patriotic in our nations? Some time ago, I read a story of a pilot who was shot down by enemy fire in the jungles of Southeast Asia. As the airman fought for his life by the side of a river alone and in agony, he waited and hoped for a rescue mission to find him. He suffered enormously. He referred later in the story to his deep love for his nation and its flag. He explained that suffering for his nation had caused him to appreciate it even more.

I mentioned in Chapter 5 that I could not sleep the two nights that followed my forty-six-hour medically induced coma. It was there that I discovered again the benefits of suffering. Lying there, I turned over and over in my mind the things that had happened to me in the previous days. I decided that the lessons I learned from suffering these wounds were too valuable to keep to myself. This book is the result of those ponderings. I "wrote" this book in my mind during those days.

Wise King Solomon said, "Wounds from a friend can be trusted" (Proverbs 27:6). God is our truest Friend. If we learn to trust His dealings with us — including the wounds — we will always find His craftsmanship capable of producing an ultimately good result. We can trust Him to work through and use even bad things for good purposes in our lives. In a world of difficulties that exist due

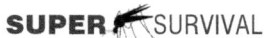

to sin, God still works for good. His ways are amazingly diverse from and superior to ours. He works His lofty and noble purposes in our lives very differently from how we would choose.

As a result of this experience and many others in life, I have resolved to seek to find the good in the wounds. That does not make the experience pleasant, but it does mean I will squeeze out of it everything worth learning. I will look for the ultimate good. Why? Because the Bible says God is working for the good in all situations. He is the Master Craftsman and can use apparent bad for ultimate good. That is the real good that makes wounds productive — and necessary.

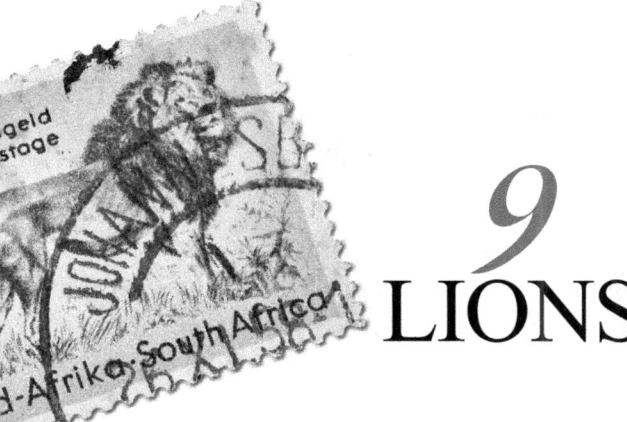

9
LIONS

We humans are fascinated with the kings of the jungle — the lions. Songs, poetry, and adventure stories are filled with lore about these majestic beasts. Tigers are bigger and up to 110 pounds (49 kilograms) heavier than lions. But it is the lion — especially the male lion — that captures the imagination of people all over the world.

Just a week before leaving Pretoria for Israel, Char and I took a three-day mini-vacation. We went to the world-famous Kruger National Park in northeastern South Africa for the very first time. This wildlife park gave us opportunities to observe many animals close-up in their natural habitat: gazelles, zebras, hippopotamuses, rhinoceroses, giraffes, warthogs, hyenas, monkeys, baboons, elephants, and wildebeests.

The highlight of those three days, however, was the day we sighted the lions. A group of us gathered in our cars on a bridge. The male was lying at the end of a log facing the bridge. He appeared in our field glasses just as magnificently poised and confident as any lion I have ever seen in a zoo, photo, painting, or in my imagination.

Not too far away, five lionesses with a number of cubs were resting and playing on a sand bar in the center of a dry river bed. One or two of the lionesses was lying on her back. Others were frolicking in playful attempts to knock the other ones over. The cubs entertained us with their playful antics. We were enthralled to be watching lions enjoying life right there in the wild.

These memories were still vivid in my mind a few weeks later in Israel as I lay on my hospital bed reflecting on my physical struggles with malaria on the night of Friday, November 5, 2010. Other memories of lions from another time eight years before also flooded in.

In 2002, while on sabbatical from lecturing at Oral Roberts University, I was teaching in South Africa. Char and I went with friends to a lion park near Johannesburg. The keepers were petting and playing with some lion cubs in a cage. They invited us to join them in the cage.

These cubs were as playful as domestic kittens. However, these "kittens" were much stronger, more stable, and coarser than the domestic cute and cuddly kittens with which we play in our homes. These cats, even though very young, were physically so firm that when we petted them there, was no soft or easy flexibility to our touch. Such impressive strength and solidity in these babies reminded us that lions are very strong animals.

We drove through the larger part of the park. We noticed the females near our vehicle were free to roam as the road led us from pride to pride. Some lionesses were lying down, and others were walking around. Some were even walking on or near the road. All of them were majestic.

In another part of that same lion park, an agitated male was pacing back and forth in a fenced enclosure. The fence was about ten feet high and made of very strong wire. Every once in a while, the large male in the enclosure would throw his weight against the fence and give out a loud roar. We eventually realized that he could hear another male not too far away. The two were challenging each other according to the natural laws of competitive male lions.

Male lions living in the comfort, safety, and provision available in a zoo can live to be twenty years old. They have no scars on their bodies and can sleep and freely move about with ease. Their viewers are satisfied with the majesty of their appearance. Their workday is short, and all their needs are met by their attendants.

But their counterparts — the males in the wild — have to really work for their living. That is, they have to work in order to stay alive. Another male lion may threaten or attack at any time. An attacker may have been raised in another pride or even his own. He could also have been the male lion's own offspring. In that case, it is likely the older male lion had earlier chased the younger one away because he was getting strong enough to challenge the older lion's dominance over the pride. Now the younger one was returning to do just that.

A male lion has scars from his battles. Either he is strong enough to maintain his position or he loses it. Typically he will be dead by the time he is ten years old. That is the law of lion country. His scars are evidence of the reality and severity of the fights between male lions throughout the wild.

As I struggled through my sickness, especially during the dark valley of weakness and great discomfort, I thought of the fights between two male lions and their struggle for dominance. Only one wins. The other lion either walks or runs away or is killed. Only one prevails; there is only one victor. My contemplations continued.

What happens when two males compete for dominion? Under what circumstances would a young male lion attack a senior male lion? When would a senior lion attack a junior lion driving the younger lion away from the pride? What kind of psychology exists in or between male lions? What are the factors that give one male lion an advantage over another? Does the fight between males depend on other factors or mostly on brute strength? What part does surprise play? A male lion can weigh 550 pounds (250 Kilograms). Is weight the major factor? Are some males more intelligent than others and, if so, in what way do they use cleverness to their advantage?

I do not have answers to all these questions that crept through my mind that night. Nevertheless, in my curiosity, I considered these matters as I meditated on a much more significant great lion fight.

I pondered a struggle between two lions which greatly affects each of our survivals. One is the devil who "prowls around like a

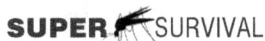

> *In His majesty, might, and power over every enemy such as sickness, sin, and weakness, He wants to show Himself strong — sometimes through you and, at other times, on your behalf.*

roaring lion looking for someone to devour" (1 Peter 5:8 NIV). The other — the Lamb that was slain and who opens the seals — is none other than the Lion of the tribe of Judah. "Do not weep! See, the Lion of the tribe of Judah, the Root of David, has triumphed" (Revelation 5:5 NIV). This great Lion manifests His majesty, authority, superiority, power, and eventual triumph over all His enemies.

Both lions want you. One wants to bless, forgive, enrich, and love you for eternity. In His majesty, might, and power over every enemy such as sickness, sin, and weakness, He wants to show Himself strong — sometimes through you and, at other times, on your behalf. He wants to give you dreams and then help you fulfill them. He wants to make life rich, abundant, full, and fulfilling for you.

The other lion wants to destroy you. He wants to deceive you so you do not realize your potential. He wants to make you doubt, fret, worry, and be so anxious about the cares of this world that you cannot possibly fulfill your dreams. He hitchhikes on normal human problems, taking advantage of the ordinary reverses of life, amplifying and expanding them beyond their actual condition. He deceptively makes problems seem much worse than they really are. In doing this, he weakens you, making you so fearful that you never try to accomplish anything lofty.

The clearest sentence describing the vast difference between what the two lions want to do to you is: "The thief comes only to steal and kill and destroy; I have come that they might have life, and have it to the full" (John 10:10 NIV).

The profound and vitally significant reality of this struggle is that we, not the lions, make the choice whether the thief or the Good Shepherd wins in our lives.

As the hours of the night of November 5, 2010 passed, I pondered the struggle between these two lions. I reflected on the difference in their character and the consequence to us as a result of our choice of which lion we follow, especially as it applied to me in my immediate circumstances.

I had been asleep for forty-six hours and now could not rest. Yet, I was glad to be conscious again. For the first time in days, I was glad to be alive. Never before had I thought things like I thought during the previous days of pain, discomfort, weakness, and helpless inability to breathe. Never before in my life had I thought, "If this is life, I do not want to live."

I realized then that the enemy had been at work. He wanted to steal my health, kill my body, and destroy the work I envision doing for God. But the Lion of the Tribe of Judah took this attack from the counterfeit lion, changed it into a victory for Himself, and used my experience to make me a better person. I am glad that I had chosen the Good Lion in early summer 1951 when I gave my life to Christ and continued to choose Him every day of my life since then. The same thing can happen for you. It can happen for any of us if we choose the right Lion.

But there is an even greater impact yet to occur in the struggle between the two lions. In the world's geopolitical arena, the eventual overthrow of the god of this age and the governments who yield to him will occur when the rightful King begins to reign on the earth.

When the Man from Nazareth was slain on the cross just outside of Jerusalem, He didn't just die for the sins of the world. He also went to hell to bring the captives out. He gives gifts to His children. He enables us to live victoriously over the world, the flesh, and the devil. He will also eventually win a smashing victory over him, breaking every chain, delivering every captive, healing every

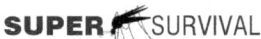

sickness, and welcoming into His eternal kingdom everyone who acknowledges Him as Savior and King.

That night, I thought not only of my victory over malaria, pneumonia, and ARDS. I also reflected on my involvement in the daily personal battle between the two lions and my on-going ministry to help others in their daily battles. I examined my participation in the eventual victory over Satan himself and my companionship with the Lion of the Tribe of Judah for eternity.

As the night passed, I rejoiced in my eventual state. I exulted in the result of the fight between two mighty lions because I knew which one would win, and that the other was only an imitation by comparison. The despair I had felt earlier dissipated while hope and courage increased.

What does this have to do with being a super-survivor?

Hope is a great power. When there is no hope, we give up and stop trying. When we have hope, we keep struggling. And because we keep striving, we keep winning. The only one who loses is the one who stops trying. My meditations on the lions gave me great hope; and in that, I am still rejoicing.

10
THE JOURNEY

Saturday, July 24, 2010, Char and I traveled from the Congos to Pretoria having completed two exhausting months of conference work. Fast-forward a couple of months. We departed from Pretoria on the evening of Monday, September 13, headed for Israel for a break. We arrived in Tiberius via Tel Aviv the following evening. The Foreword and Chapter 1 provide the details of the days leading up to my hospitalization.

This part of the book chronicles the days after my hospitalization. We've woven together the photos, x-rays, and well wishes from those who love and support us and our work.

It was very disappointing to have to cancel/postpone our five weeks of seminars scheduled in Rwanda. As you can tell from this book, I do not give up easily. Nevertheless, the brethren there wrote a number of encouraging notes to us.

As you look at the x-rays, you'll notice the color change. Cloudiness or white areas represent fluid and mucus. The more cloudy or white the area, the more fluid and mucus that was present. You will be able to see the progression as my lungs filled up more and more during the first several days. Observe the progress as the medications and the power of God reversed the process during the following days.

I've included the dates on the x-rays. They will help you appreciate how quickly this occurred. The whole process was over in just twelve days.

Saturday, October 30

We arrived about 9:30 a.m. at the emergency unit of the Baruch Padeh Medical Center in Poriya on our way to worship nearby. We were scheduled to depart on October 31 for a conference series in Rwanda that ran from November 1 to December 6. After extensive blood tests, an x-ray, and being given a preliminary diagnosis of malaria, I was admitted to the internal medicine unit of the hospital. I seemed to be okay as I sat up and chatted with visitors.

The prayers, encouragement, and support we received from family and friends around the world during my illness and recovery were much more than we could have imagined. We are blessed, humbled, and full of gratitude to all who prayed for us and wrote to us during this time. In many ways, the victory in which we now walk is theirs — yours — as well.

We could never be able to share all the e-mails and Facebook posts that came our way. And it has been painful to have to be selective. For all who wrote, please rest assured that we will be eternally grateful for you.

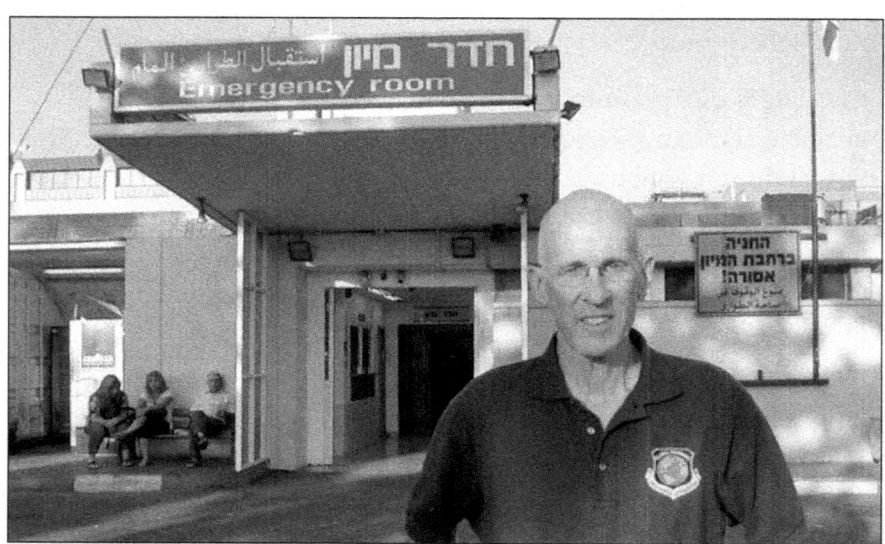

Emergency Entrance. This photo was taken the next day after release from the hospital when I am clean-shaven again. This is the entrance to our adventure in the Poriya Hospital via the emergency room.

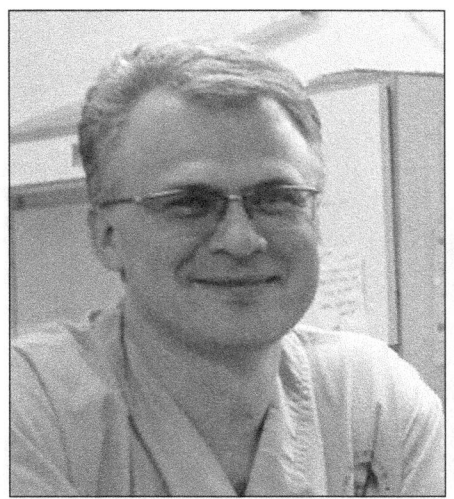 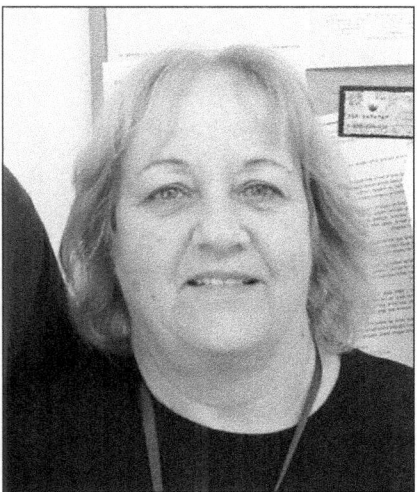

Emergency Technician (left). This technician has exceedingly nimble fingers and good dexterity. He took six samples of blood in about one minute.

Original Receptionist (right). Ruth is the kind, English-speaking lady who helped us with emergency room entrance procedures on October 30.

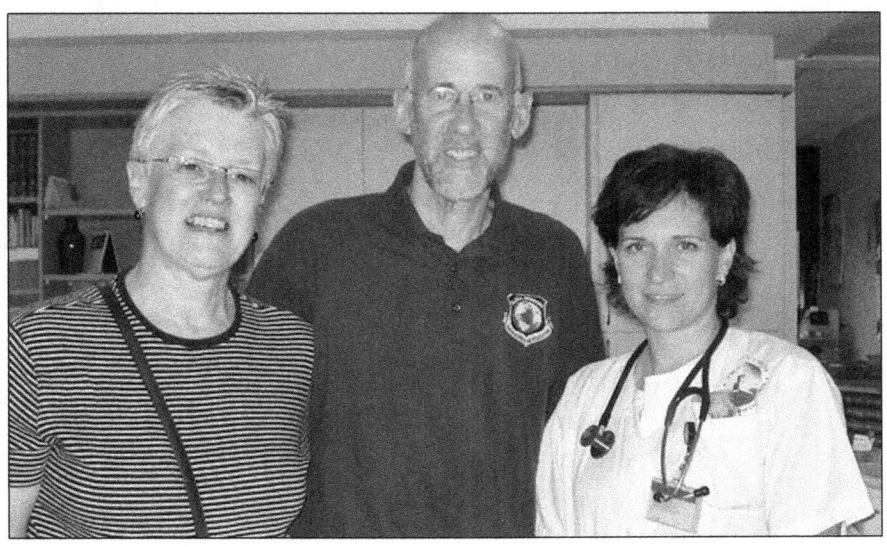

Char and I with the Emergency Doctor. This was taken the day of my release from the hospital. This Russian doctor served in the emergency ward the day I arrived. She was later stationed in the internal medicine ward where I was when I was released.

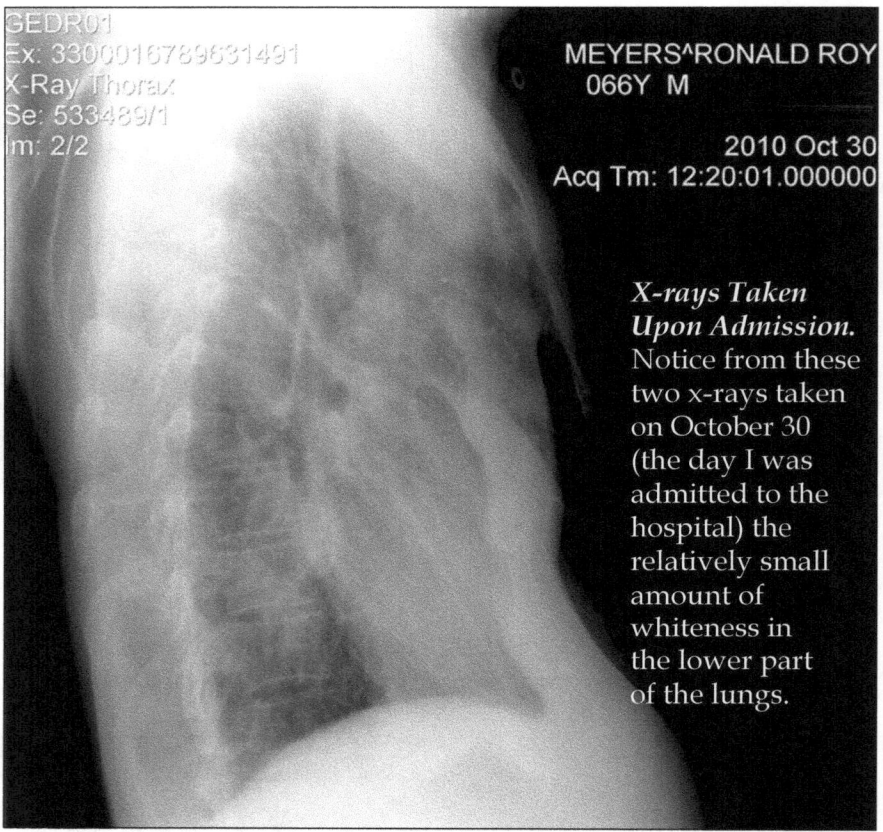

X-rays Taken Upon Admission. Notice from these two x-rays taken on October 30 (the day I was admitted to the hospital) the relatively small amount of whiteness in the lower part of the lungs.

A note from Ananias in Rwanda:

> Dear Char and Ron,
>
> We are very touched by Ron's health situation but the will of God will turn to reality.
>
> There is no fear or discouragement because we strongly believe that our God is in control. We are praying for you all. Let's wait for the good will of God our Father. I don't personally have any problem with getting the convention postponed. I believe God has a different and sweet plan/will for all of us. We will see the tremendous treasure that God reserves for us in the future. Surely we will love it.

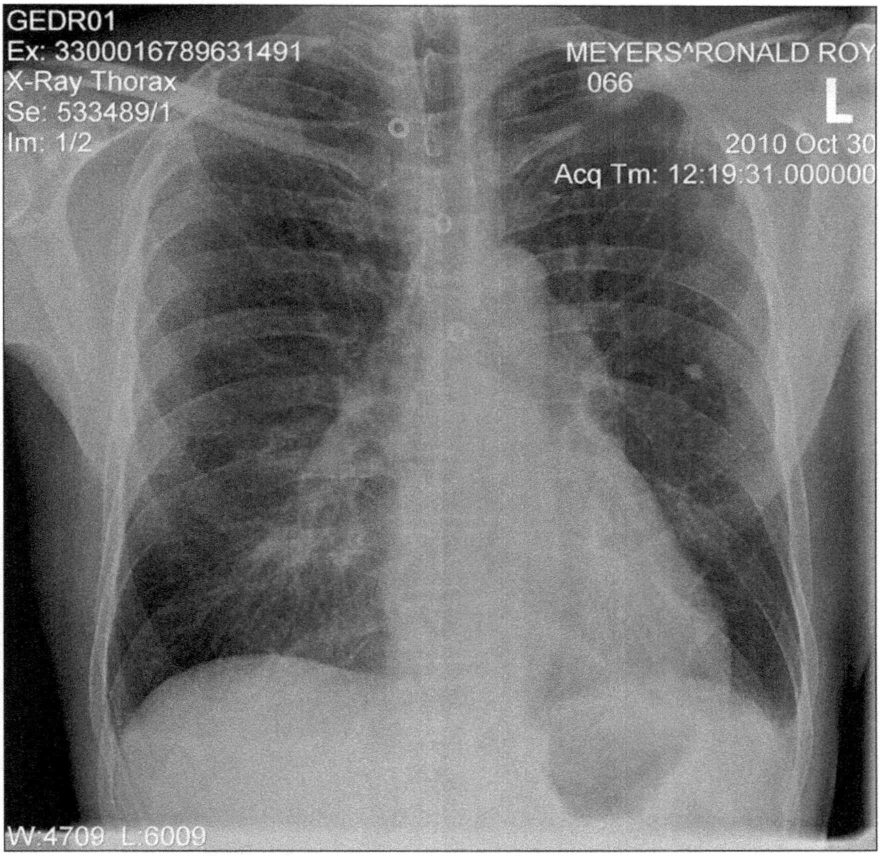

Ananias also sent the words of the following hymn:

> O love that will not let me go,
> I rest my weary soul on thee;
> I give thee back the life I owe,
> That in thine ocean depths its flow
> May richer, fuller be.
>
> O joy that seekest me through pain,
> I cannot close my heart to thee;
> I trace the rainbow through the rain,
> And feel the promise is not vain
> That morn shall tearless be.

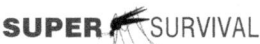

Sunday, October 31

I spent the day declining in strength and the ability to breathe. By evening, I was gasping for each breath and breathing very quickly. Attempts to affix a mask to my face brought terror to me. I really worked to cooperate, but I was not receiving enough air. I was moved to the intensive cardiac care unit (ICCU) where I was given oxygen and then morphine to calm me. I slept through the night. Throughout the night, Char made several calls to the ICCU. Each time, nurses reported I was resting.

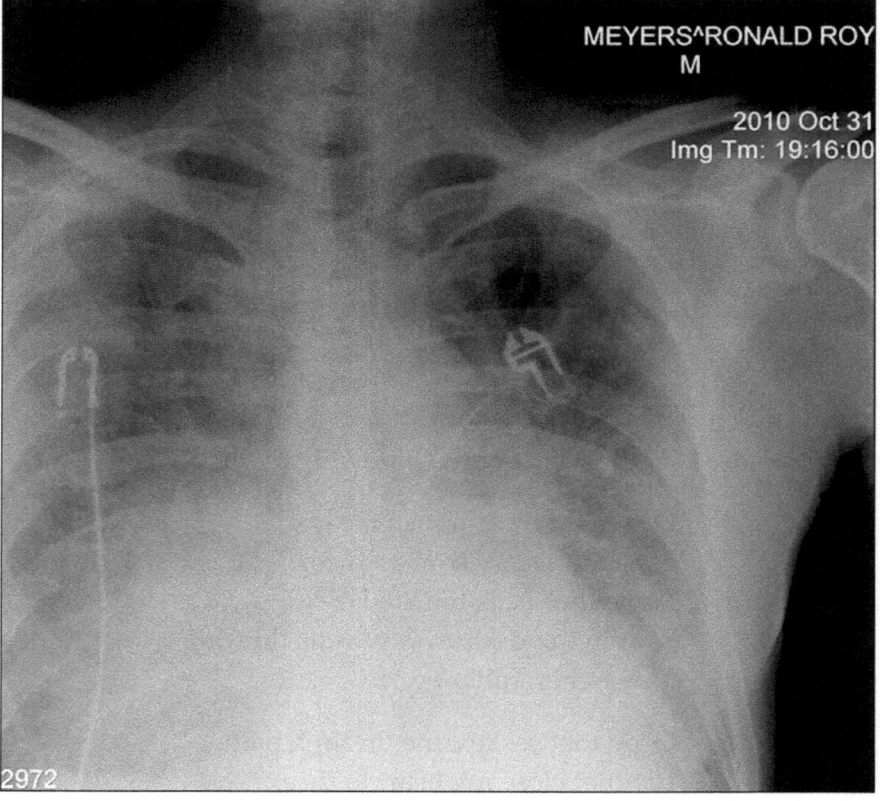

Evidence of My Deteriorating Condition. Notice the increased amount of whiteness on October 31 (the second day).

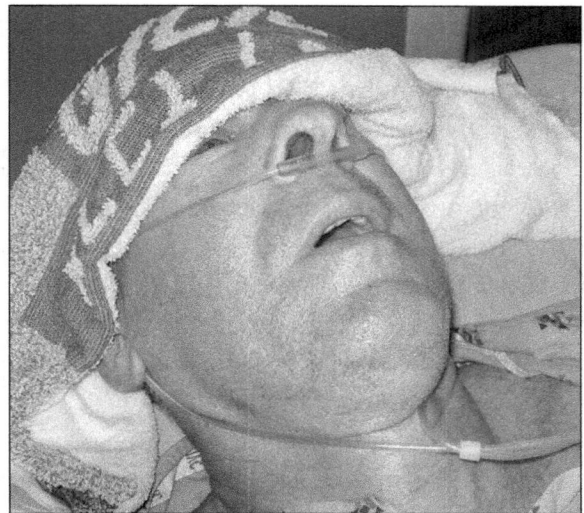

Before Coma. I have been diagnosed with malaria but do not yet know that I have extensive pneumonia in both lungs that later precipitates acute respiratory distress syndrome (ARDS). I am seriously ill, and my condition is deteriorating.

And from other brothers and sisters in Rwanda:

> Dear Char,
>
> Greetings in Christ's name. I hope God is hearing our prayers. We are together with you though we are far physically. But be assured of our prayers. May we know the progress of how Dr. Ron is feeling? I hope we may one day see him face to face! May the hand of God be upon you all.
>
> Mike

We also received many e-mails from friends in other African nations outside of Rwanda:

> I have called my family and my team and pastor friends, and we are praying for that mighty man of God. God is his Boss and is in control. Please, Char, let me know how the change is coming in his body.
>
> Pierre

Monday, November 1

In the morning, I seemed to be improving and was moved to the intensive care unit (ICU) so they could continue to monitor my vital signs. This day, three x-rays were taken: two in the morning and one in the evening. As the afternoon progressed, I struggled more and more to breathe. The doctor informed me that in addition to pneumonia, I also had acute respiratory distress syndrome (ARDS). I called Char to tell her. About 8:30 that evening after my visitors who had come to pray for me left, I was told I would be put to sleep and that I would wake up with ventilator tubes in my throat. I went into a medically induced coma for about forty-six hours. During the second hour of the coma, I experienced on-again, off-again ventricle tachycardia — in my case, a heart rate of 200 beats per minute.

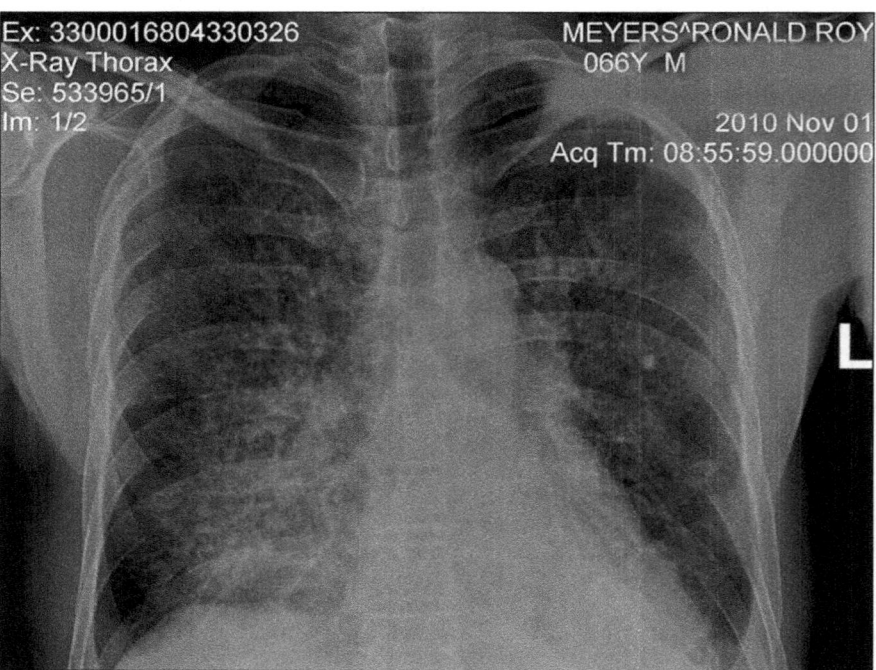

The Third Day. This x-ray was taken the evening of November 1. It indicates a significant increase of fluid and mucus gathered during just that one day.

"But if the Spirit of Him who raised Jesus from the dead dwells in you, He who raised Christ from the dead will also give life to your mortal bodies through His Spirit who dwells in you."

Lord, you can do ANYTHING ...

"And ye shall serve the Lord your God, and he shall bless thy bread, and thy water; and I will take sickness away from the midst of thee."

The church is praying for you all ... the Lord is doing what only He can do ... We stand with you.

Innocent

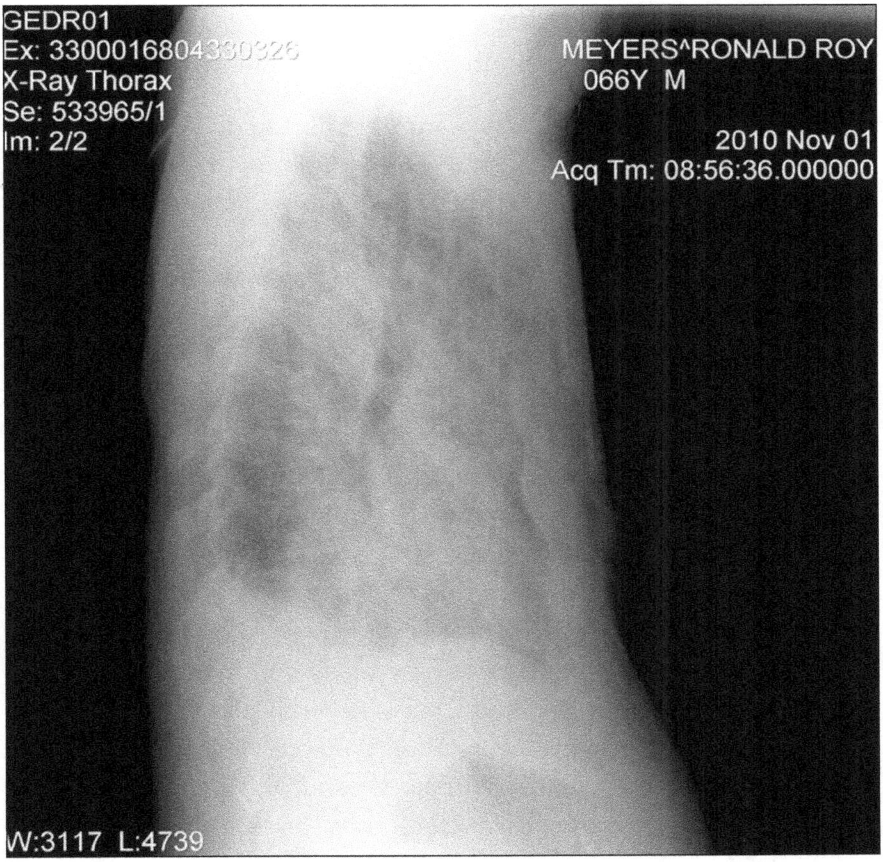

Increasing Whiteness in the Lungs. This x-ray was taken just before 9:00 a.m. on the morning of November 1, the third day in the hospital.

The prayer of the saints here is that Papa will fully recover and be on his feet again. Mama, the Lord is your strength and support. All will be well in Jesus' name.
Joshua

Messages too numerous to count kept coming.

Prayer to our Almighty God arose from around the world on our behalf. Here are just a few of those words of blessing. We are sorry we cannot print all of them.

Char—

I really had a good chat with Marilyn, and we prayed hard for Ron. Sterling is concerned too.

Love John (Char's brother John in Maryland)

Lord, as I sit here at my computer, I lift up to you Ron and Char Meyers. Even though you know their needs even better than I do, I pray that you will continue to intervene in their lives. In your capacity as the Great Physician, I pray that you will cast out that army of parasites from Ron's body. It is also my prayer that you will not allow the evil one or his angels to interfere or discourage Ron or Char. We know of your promise to "never leave us or forsake us" and that "nothing can separate us from You." However, in our human condition, we can become discouraged, angry, or confused. Therefore, I pray that you would continue to reveal yourself to Char during this period of Ron's illness in a powerful and dynamic way so that none of these negative feelings will permeate her in any way. Surround both Ron and Char with your powerful love as well as your divine healing. We all love you, Lord, and we give You all of the honor and praise. I lift up this prayer in the powerful name of Jesus. Amen.
Dick

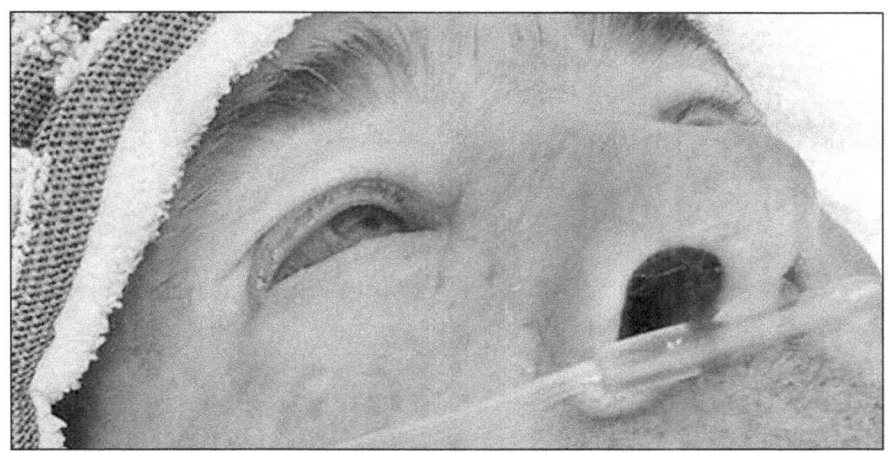

Before the Coma. The distress my body was experiencing is apparent in my eyes.

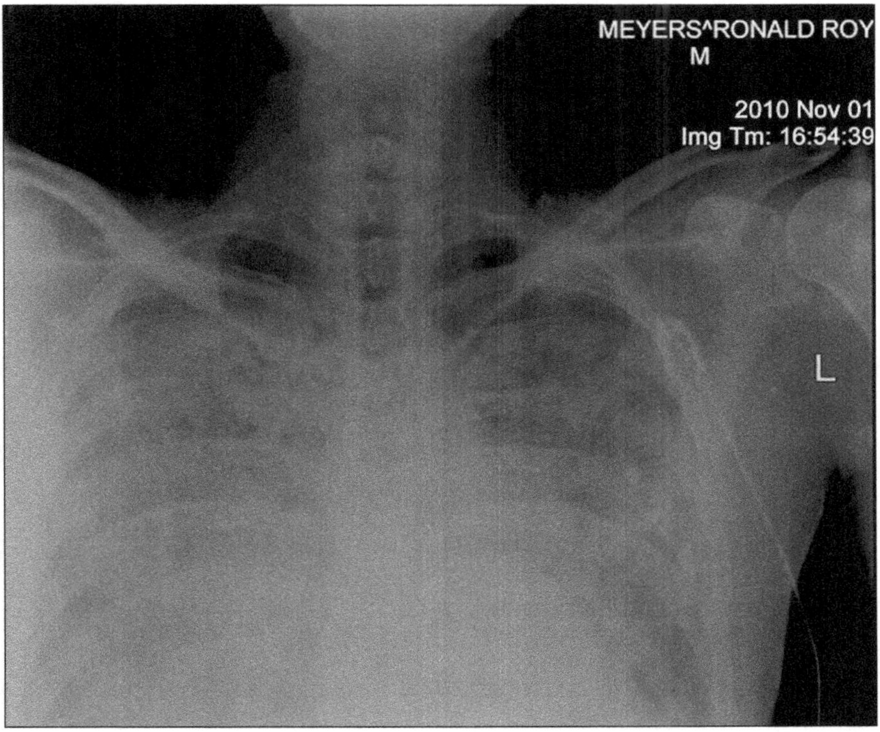

Still More Whiteness in the Lungs. This x-ray was taken the evening of November 1 (the third day in the hospital). It indicates a significant increase of fluid and mucus gathered during just that one day.

Tuesday, November 2

My drugged condition left me with only one memory from this day: I thought I was in a military hospital and was being held in bed by a net attached to my head. In reality, I was simply lying in the bed with multiple needles in both arms to allow for intravenous feeding, administering of various drugs, and periodic blood extraction. I also had tubes in my nose and throat. When Char talked with the doctor midday, he said if our sons wanted to visit with their father, they could come. Then she asked, "Is he good?" He answered, "He is better, but he is not good." He did not mention my ventricle tachycardia. Based on this information, our two sons, Dan and Joel, decided that Dan would make the trip representing both of them. Joel prepared to come later if it became necessary.

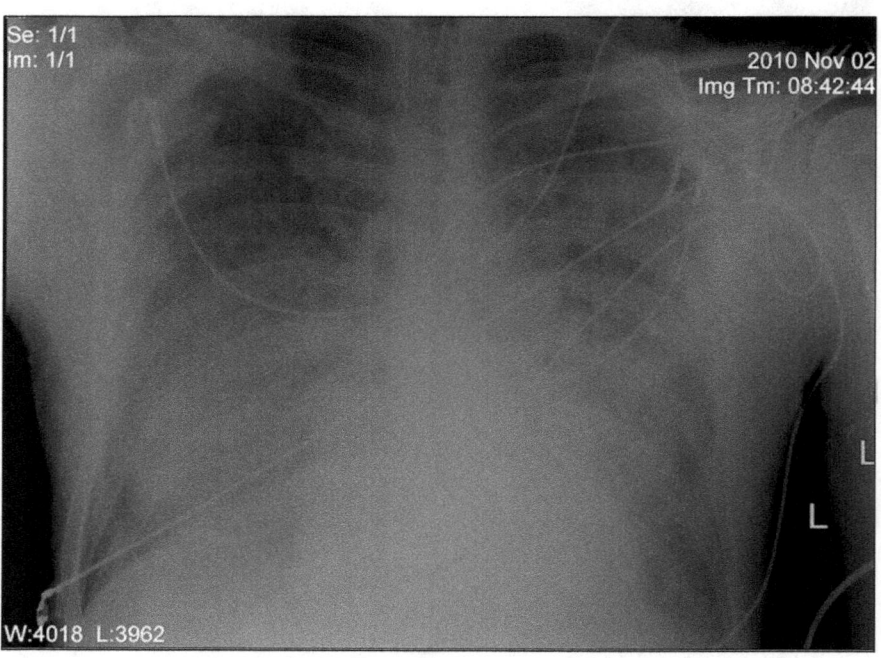

Malaria Appears to Be Winning the Battle. This x-ray taken the morning of November 2 (the fourth day in the hospital) illustrates the increase of fluid and mucus accumulated during the night of November 1 and 2. I was in an induced coma on this day.

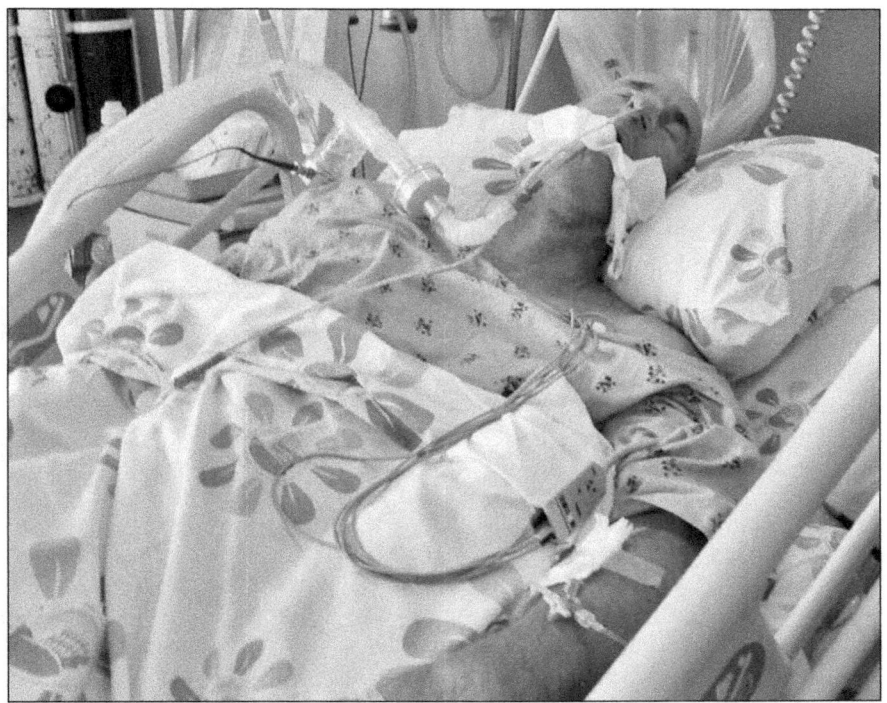

In a Coma with a Ventilator. The ventilator in my throat forced oxygenated air into my bronchial tubes for ninety-six hours. For the first forty-six hours, I was unconscious in an induced coma. During the first hour of the coma, my heart went in and out of ventricular tachycardia with a pulse of 200 heartbeats per minute.

> Know you are surrounded with the love of God. I pray that you can feel a strong presence of God in the room. We love you.
>
> Annie

> My dear Char,
>
> How I wish I could be beside you literally to support and care. Please know that is my heart for you, as you two struggle with the enormity of this crisis. "Lord, get those boys to their mom and dad quickly and without logistical problems. Amen."
>
> Connie

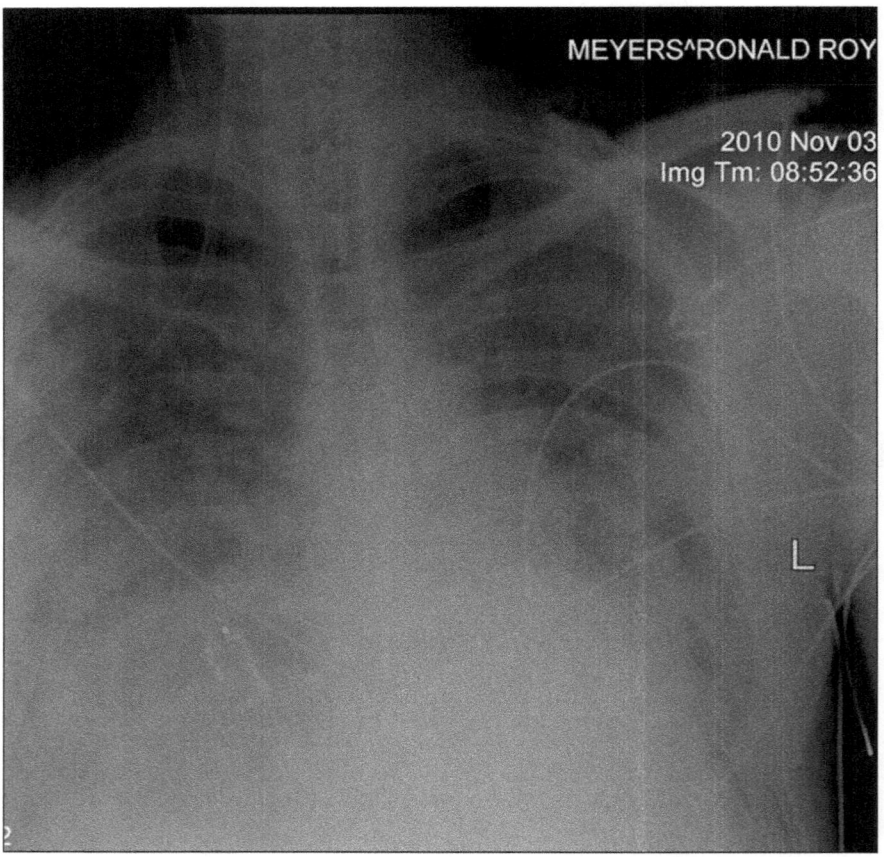

My Illness Is Still Progressing. This x-ray was taken the morning of November 3 (the fifth day in the hospital). It shows the malaria and pneumonia depositing still more fluid and mucus into my lungs. I remained in a coma and was unaware this x-ray was being taken.

Wednesday, November 3

Our son Dan arrived from Canada that evening and stood by my bedside along with Char. It was then, after forty-six hours in a coma, that I began to awaken only slightly as Dan spoke to me and I recognized his voice. In this semi-conscious state — they told me later — I could only communicate by flickering my eyebrows or moving my left hand. Meanwhile, I also had to fight to keep from going crazy with the ventilator tickling my throat.

The Scriptures were especially encouraging and uplifting. This excerpt from Psalm 121 was sent by Ron's brother-in-law, John:

> "The Lord is your guardian;
> The Lord is your shade at your right hand.
>
> By day the sun cannot harm you,
> Nor the moon by night.
>
> The Lord will guard you from all evil,
> Will always guard your life;
>
> The Lord will guard your coming and going
> Both now and forever."

Then he added the following thoughts:

> I see some similarities in Ron's life to that of the Apostle Paul ... both exceptional men of God, well-traveled teachers, who hunger to see the lost restored, and now may share the same "thorn in the flesh."
>
> If this is out of line, please let me know ... have you ever felt that it might be time to "put down the passport and pick up the pen?" Begin writing curriculum/letters to pastors and churches that will help them continue to grow and expand their outreach ... to travel closer to home where perhaps the health risks are not so great. This has been on my heart for several days so I just thought I'd share it with you.
>
> Blessings on you both.
> John

My response:

> Thanks for your deep concern, John. We believe we must keep on going as long as we can.
> Ron

I see the value of John's suggestion.

Thursday, November 4

At midday, following Dan's lead, we tried to communicate by my responding to each letter of the alphabet as Dan attempted to get information from me. It seems to me that this day was a turning point. At noon, I was responding to the medication. By evening, I moved my arms.

I'm glad Dan is coming. He can be your "rock" for awhile and give you a giant hug. He is really good at that.
Shannon

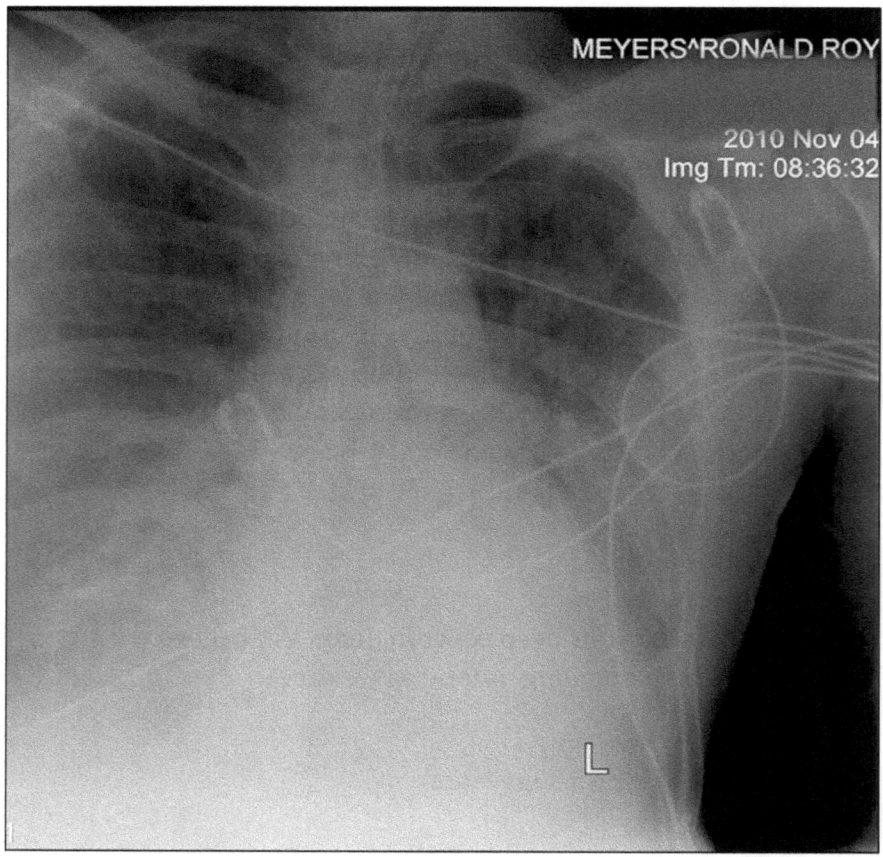

Day Six in the Hospital. Taken the morning of November 4, this photo seems to indicate a slight recession of the whiteness.

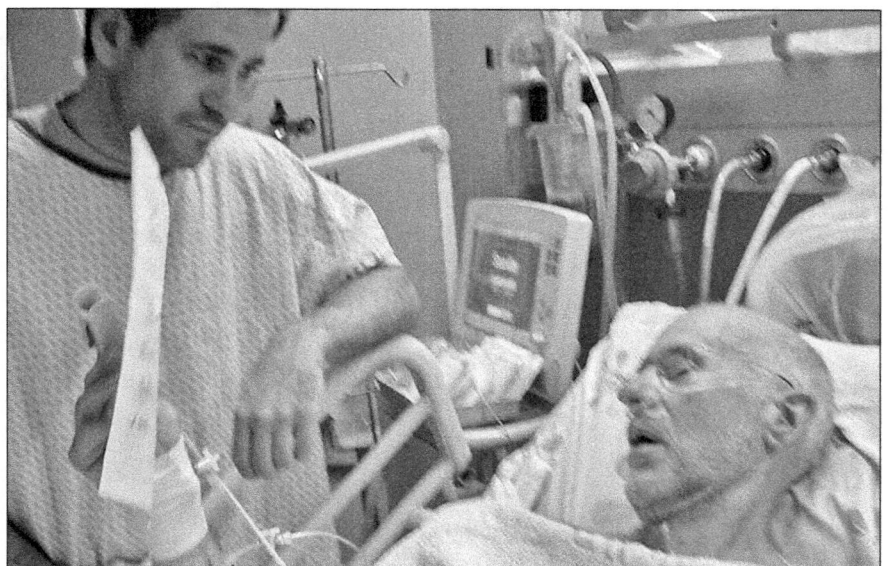

Dan and Dad. After becoming conscious and before I could talk again, Dan and I worked hard to communicate via a sheet of paper with the letters of the alphabet on it. You can see that paper here.

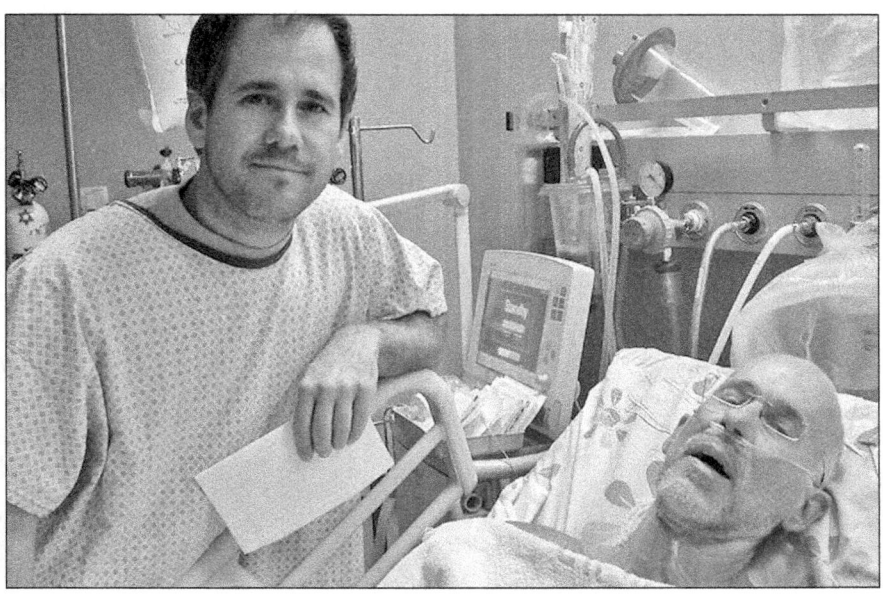

My Son, My Encourager. Dan's visit was a tremendous source of strength to both Char and me. He also represented our son Joel and his family, and I was very much aware of that the whole time he was there.

Friday, November 5

The ventilator was removed at 3:00 p.m. I was told I would begin recovery and therapy the next day. I began to talk again with a very raspy voice as soon as the ventilator was removed.

> Char,
>
> Cherie and I continue to pray through this with you and Ron. We didn't get the full picture at first. Thank God you had not left Israel. We know Ron is getting good care there.
>
> Barry
>
> Just saw the news of Ron in ICCU, and Bern and I are praying for you both!
>
> Pamela

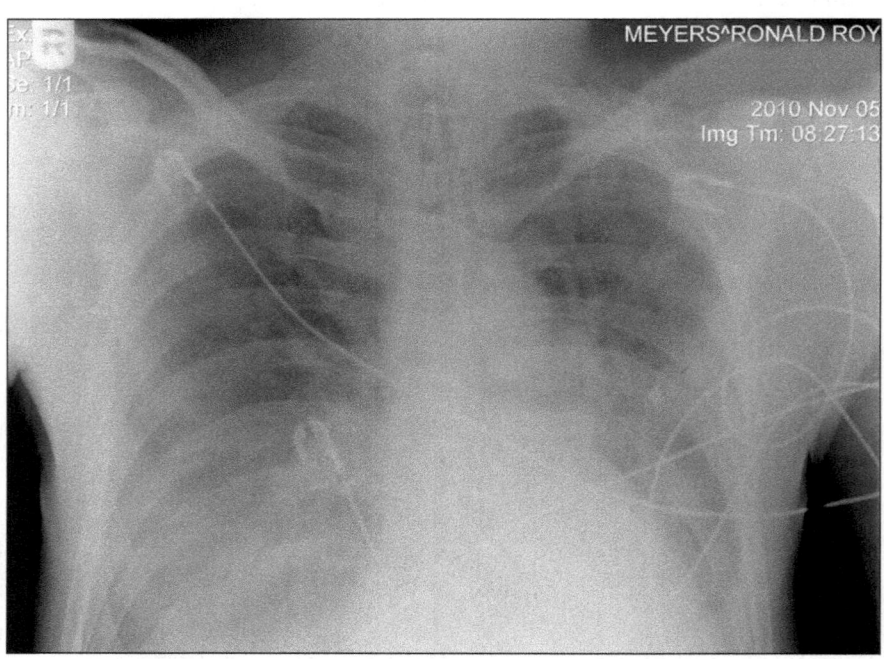

Day Seven in the Hospital. This x-ray was taken the morning of November 5. It shows slightly less accumulation than was present on November 4.

After Char reported on Facebook, "RESPIRATOR IS OUT AND RON'S TALKING! We are dancing here ... join us!" there were other messages of praise and ongoing support.

> Nothing less than awesome! To God be the glory and praise. Tomorrow he will be talking like a machine, ready to go! What an experience for you and Dan to witness.
> Charlene

> The greatest news of the year. PTL! God is awesome!
> Andrew

> We are so thrilled that the Lord has brought you and Ron through this. He is indeed our Healer. We are praying with you all for complete health and wholeness.
> Rich and Su

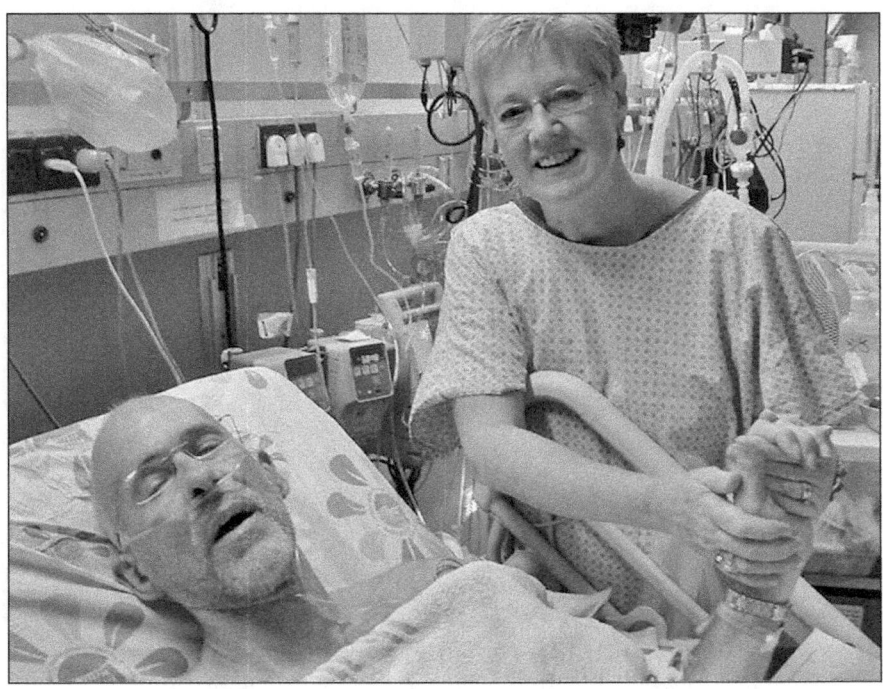

Ron and Char. Char almost became a widow. In this picture, you can see I had turned the corner, and it appeared that I was on the mend.

Saturday, November 6

Physical therapy began with breathing exercises. It took me six minutes, assisted by the nurses, to get out of bed; and then I sat in a chair for about five hours. My intestinal movements began.

After coming out of the medically induced coma, I informed people that I intended to write this book and shared the general thoughts it would contain. So many responded.

> Ron and Char:
>
> Praise God that He saw you through! We definitely will want to read the e-book. We now will be praying more intelligently for you and for your complete recovery.
>
> Larry and Ruthann

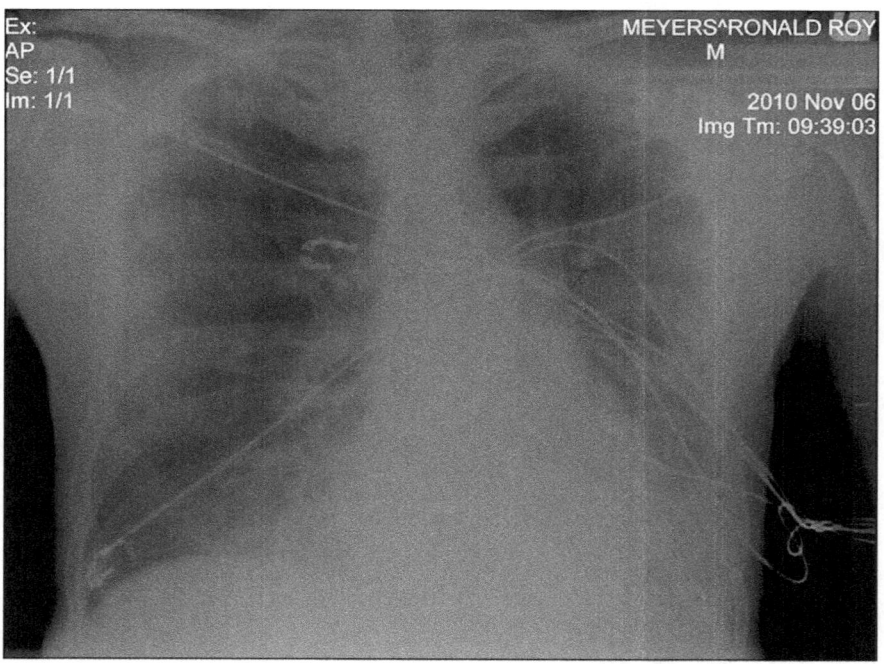

Day Eight in the Hospital. Taken the morning of November 6, this x-ray shows a clearer indication that the pneumonia is receding. God and the medicine are winning. I got out of bed and sat up for the first time later this morning.

Hi Ron.

Three cheers for the Lion of Judah!!! He does great work!!! Your beautiful view should be restful. I know taking it easy is not in your makeup, so I'm glad you're willing to obey doctor's orders. Having an e-book to do will help pass the time. I look forward to the chapters.

Kay

Dear Ron and Char,

It was so wonderful to hear from you with the good news of God's healing power in your body. You truly have experienced physical suffering to the very limit, but God was faithful and is bringing you through day by day with His strength ... Now we need to give God equal time in praising and thanking Him for His goodness and mercy to you ... We love you both dearly.

Aunt Chloris and Uncle Floyd

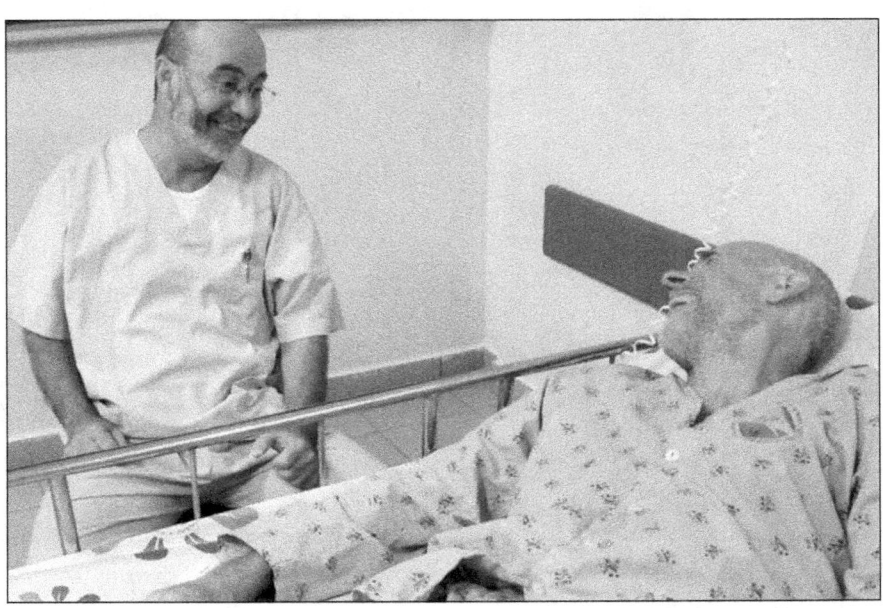

Ron and the ICU Doctor. This ICU doctor took a special interest in my case. Here we are chatting in the internal medicine unit the day after I was released from the ICU.

> **Sunday, November 7**
>
> I received my second lesson in physical therapy exercise. I got out of bed in only one minute and sat in a chair for about six hours.

Ron and Char,

I just got your e-mail, and I could not be more encouraged by its contents. Praise the Lord! We were in much agony of soul in prayer for you, and the news is a definite answer to prayer. I'll be looking forward to reading your book that catalogues all your experiences and lessons.

Trevor

Day Nine in the Hospital. This x-ray was taken on the morning of November 7. To my untrained eye, it does not show any appreciable improvement over the previous day. But to the trained eye of the radiologist and physicians, it evidently showed enough improvement that I continued my recovery program of breathing exercises and getting out of bed.

Thanking Jesus for holding your heart in His hand!!! He always does ... And God "breathed into his nostrils the breath of life and he became a living soul." And Jesus breathed on them and said, "Receive the Holy Spirit ... As the Father sent me into the world, so I send you into the world." May the "ruach/pneuma" (breath) of Jesus be the breath in Ron's lungs!

When the woman reached out for Jesus, she thought in her heart that just a touch of the hem of his garment could make her every whit whole. Right NOW, many who are the very members of His body, of His flesh, and of His bone are now being touched with Ron's need for healing. That is more intimate to the Eternal Giver of Life than just the hem of His earthly garment that gave her perfect soundness that day. May this day mark a miracle of healing in Ron's body. The miraculous health-imparting life of Jesus flows amongst us as we agree in prayer for him to be every whit whole!!!!

Love you guys and grateful for your example of faith and faithfulness.

Ray

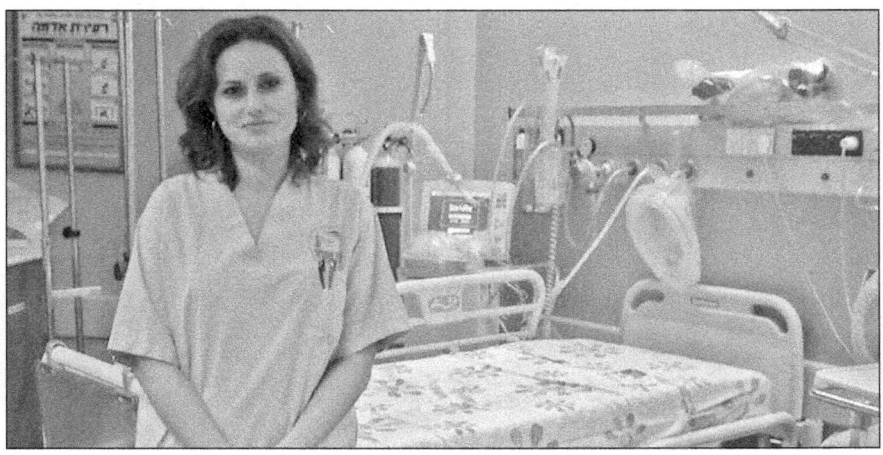

One of My ICU Nurses. I have not yet decided if my nurses were angels or human. They were wonderful agents of healing for which I will always be grateful.

Monday, November 8

I was still in the ICU. I met my third physical therapist and did more serious breathing exercises. I moved back to the internal medicine unit and began to walk to the nurses' desk about fourteen meters from my bed.

> Many in Gettysburg, PA are praying for your family ... so glad Dan is with you ... Ron is such a crusader for Jesus. He has so much more to give for the Kingdom.
> Wendy

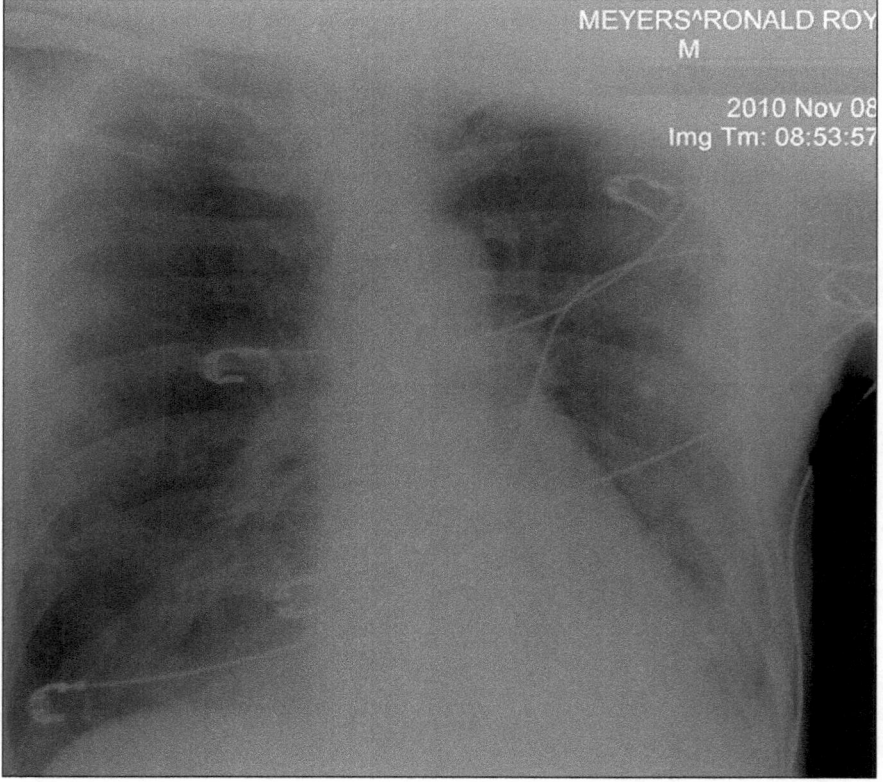

The Final X-ray. This was taken the morning of November 8 (the tenth day in the hospital and two days before my release). It reveals lungs that have cleared up even more than the previous two days. I began to walk on this day.

Our daughter-in-law, Elizabeth, wrote out Psalm 91 for us. What a blessing this psalm is.

Psalm 91 (NIV)

Whoever dwells in the shelter of the Most High
>will rest in the shadow of the Almighty.

I will say of the Lord, "He is my refuge and my fortress,
>my God, in whom I trust."

Surely he will save you from the fowler's snare
>and from the deadly pestilence.

He will cover you with his feathers,
>and under his wings you will find refuge;
>his faithfulness will be your shield and rampart.

You will not fear the terror of night,
>nor the arrow that flies by day,
>nor the pestilence that stalks in the darkness,
>nor the plague that destroys at midday.

A thousand may fall at your side,
>ten thousand at your right hand,
>but it will not come near you.

You will only observe with your eyes
>and see the punishment of the wicked.

If you say, "The Lord is my refuge,"
>and you make the Most High your dwelling,
>no harm will overtake you,
>no disaster will come near your tent.

For he will command his angels concerning you
>to guard you in all your ways;
>they will lift you up in their hands,
>so that you will not strike your foot against a stone.

You will tread on the lion and the cobra;
>you will trample the great lion and the serpent.

"Because he loves me," says the Lord, "I will rescue him;
>I will protect him, for he acknowledges my name.

He will call on me, and I will answer him;
>I will be with him in trouble,
>I will deliver him and honor him.

With long life I will satisfy him
>and show him my salvation."

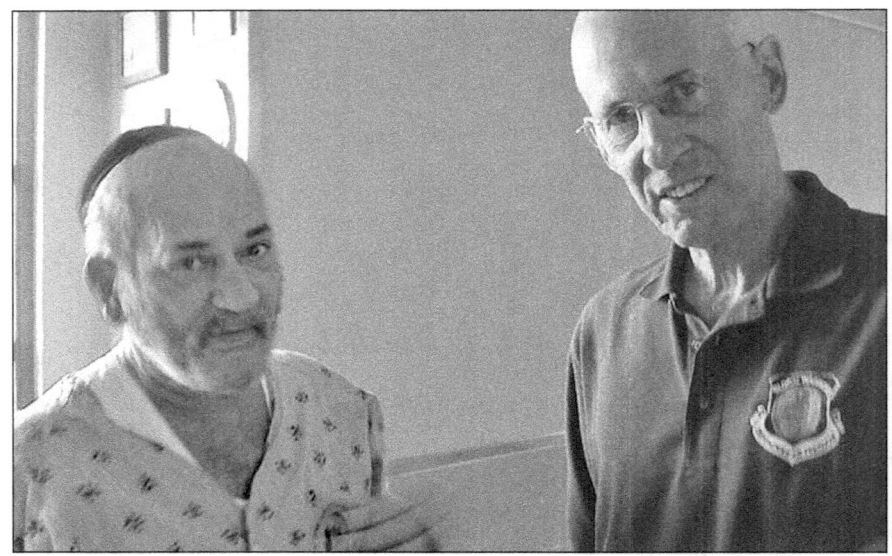

Another ICU Patient and Ron. The day I left the ICU, I struggled over to this man's side of the room to greet him and wish him well. Three days later, when I was out of the hospital, I returned to greet him again.

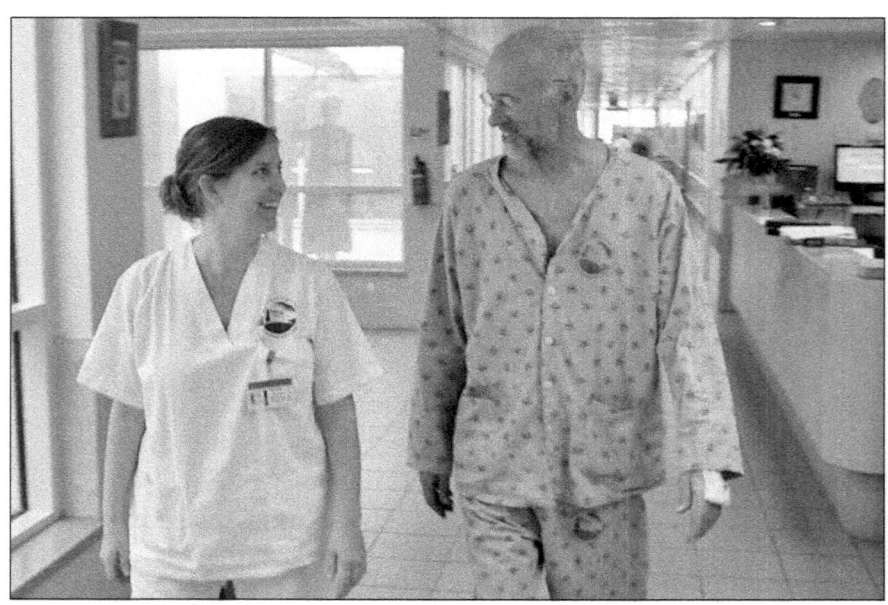

Third Therapist and Ron. Of the three therapists mentioned in Chapter 2 who worked with me, this one pushed me the most. She earned my genuine appreciation and respect for her and her profession.

Tuesday, November 9

I was told I would be released that day, but the medical release forms were not complete. I was asked to stay for another day. I learned later that the doctor wanted to observe me one more day. During that night, Dan traveled from Tiberius to Tel Aviv. He departed for Canada at 6:30 a.m. the next morning.

Dear Char,

Know that Barry and I are keeping vigil with you. I am checking my e-mail several times a day to keep up with how things are going. Keep the news coming. I am so glad you have a new congregation/family of two weeks to stand by you ... God is good.

Love, Cherie

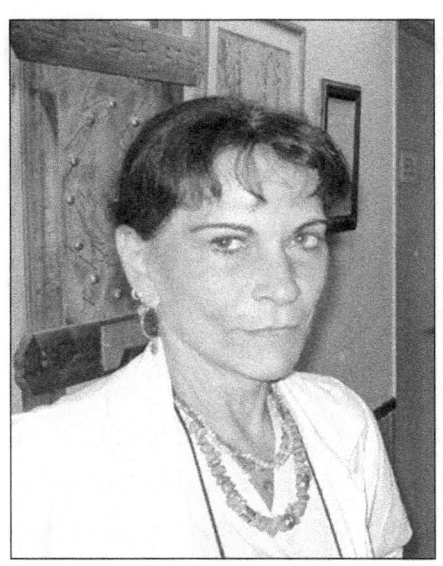
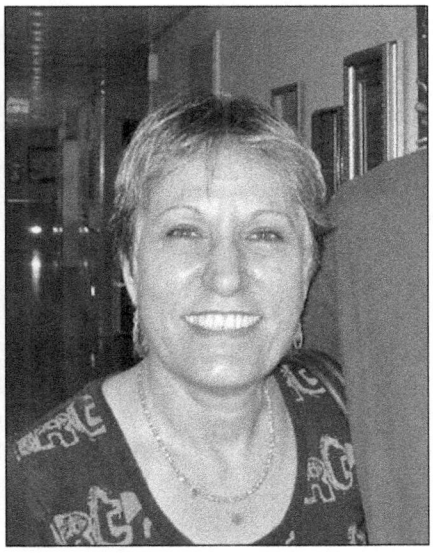

One of My ICU Doctors (left). This wonderful lady along with her two colleagues had advanced training in emergency and intensive care medicines. All three of them were highly competent professionals.

One of My ICU Nurses (right). This senior nurse in the ICU required me to hold to strictly good patient behavior. She is one of the angels who saved my life.

You are in good care at Poriya Hospital ... some of the best docs in Israel are there. I am grateful your son is with you and wish we were there with you as well.
Vicky

Hi Char!

I am so sorry for what you are going through, but the LORD will see you and Ron through this. As I was reading the comments on here, the only thing I was thinking was this is only a "weapon" of the enemy. We have to remember that NO WEAPON FORMED AGAINST US WILL PROSPER. We are believing for a COMPLETE recovery ... and an awesome testimony from him!

Love ya! Beth

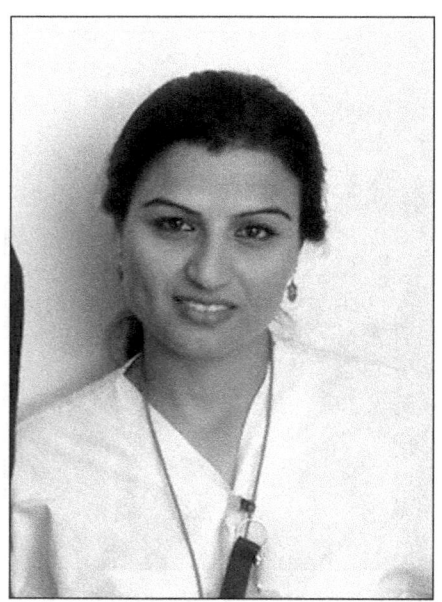 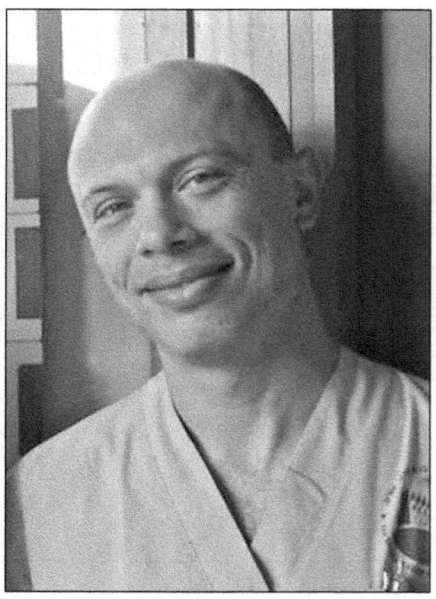

More ICU Nurses. The nurse on the left served me both in the intensive care unit and also in the internal medicine ward when I moved there. The nurse on the right was nicknamed (by himself) the Russian Mafia. He was a skilled professional who attended me carefully one entire night.

God is an awesome God, and His hand is on Ron.
Jan

Char,
Tell Ron the world seems to be praying for him. Take serious care of yourself, Char. The caretakers must be strengthened (notice I said strengthened, not strong). We love you.
Sandy, Bob, and Ben

God sees what we cannot. He is steering the ship and is in TOTAL CHARGE!
Lois and Everett

Some friends of ours in France en route back to Pretoria, South Africa wrote:

As we were driving back to Paris yesterday ... this verse came to me that I believe is for you and Ron. "They that trust in the Lord shall be as Mount Zion which shall not be moved but abideth forever ... as the mountains are around Jerusalem so the Lord is round about his people both now and forever."
Rest well.
Love,
Pat and Gerald

Still more blessings came after I was released from hospital.

Dearest Pastors Ron and Char,
We praise our Father with you to hear of His healing power in your life! We will continue to ask Him to heal you back to health quickly and are eager to read the valuable lessons that Father has taught you through this time. :) Much love and blessings to you both!
Linda and Daniel

> **Wednesday, November 10**
>
> I was told about ovale malaria (malaria eggs which would produce yet another generation of malaria) that remained in my liver. I received careful instruction to continue to take the ovale malaria medicine for thirteen more days. I was released from the hospital about 7:00 p.m.

From your experiences we will all benefit, but may you receive the broadest range of benefits that only God has the pleasure of conceiving for you and your future.
Sandy, Bob, and Ben

The name of Ron Meyers has become famous … we look forward to his coming to Rwanda soon so we can see the man God saved from death!
Mike

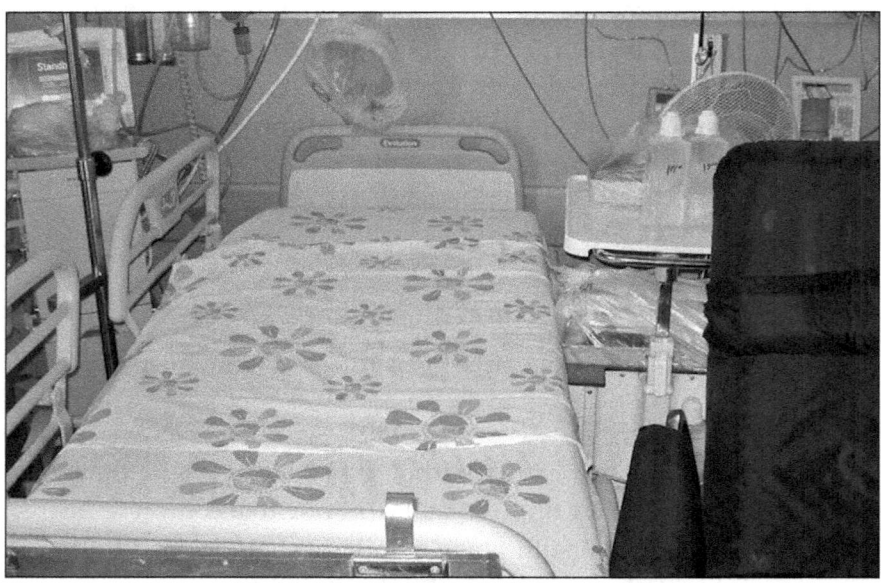

The Empty Bed. "He is not here; he has risen" (Luke 24:6 NIV). "And if the Spirit of him who raised Jesus from the dead is living in you, he who raised Christ from the dead will also give life to your mortal bodies because of his Spirit who lives in you" (Romans 8:11 NIV).

Thursday, November 11

Char and I returned to the hospital to receive the supply of ovale malaria medicine. We also took photos of and with hospital personnel in a personal victory march. My body was very weak and I had to walk at a slow pace, but I was well. I continued my breathing and walking exercises during that walk and also later in our apartment.

I concluded that I had a choice: I could either begin to take it easy in life; or, if I wanted to, I could again use free weights, stretch, walk, eventually run, and become strong in body again. I decided to pursue the latter.

> May this "down" time be a preparation for the next spiritual "race" for the Meyers.
> Connie

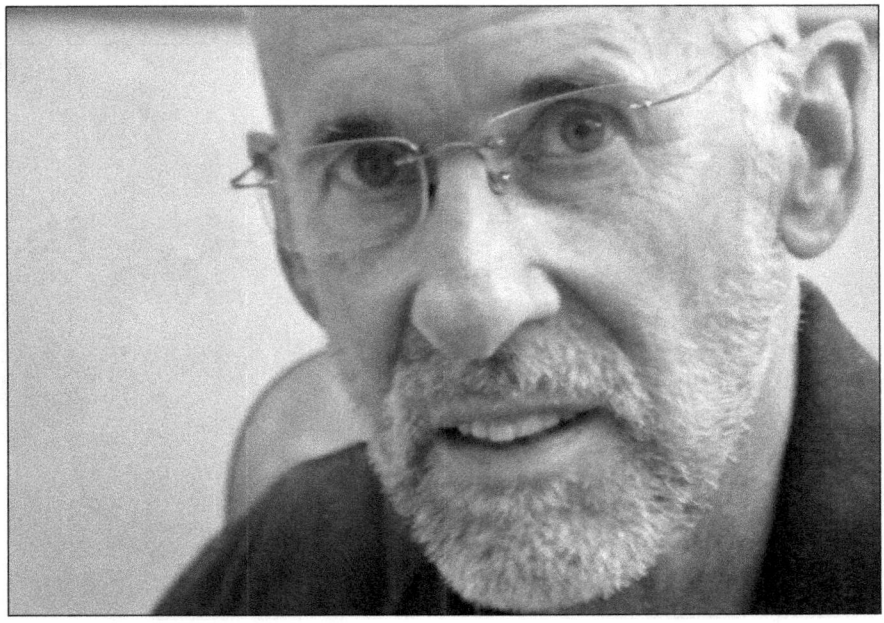

Ron with a Twelve-Day Growth of Beard. I shaved it off the next day after being released from the hospital, but I felt quite in style even with an unplanned beard of twelve days growth.

Dear Ron,

Who would have thought many years ago ... that these many years later God would allow me to be in a position and capacity to partner with you and Char and be a part of your prayer team. It has been humbling for your army of prayer warriors, I am sure, and for me. I have felt drawn to my knees and called to fast. I value your friendship so much and will keep asking God to strengthen you and restore you to the ministry you love so much.

Continue to follow doctor's orders, Ron. I know your will and strength will return, we claim it in His name. I have both you and Char daily in my prayers and my ear opened to any needs or issues that God speaks. Take care and remember, you are loved, cared for, and constantly in my prayers.

Charlene

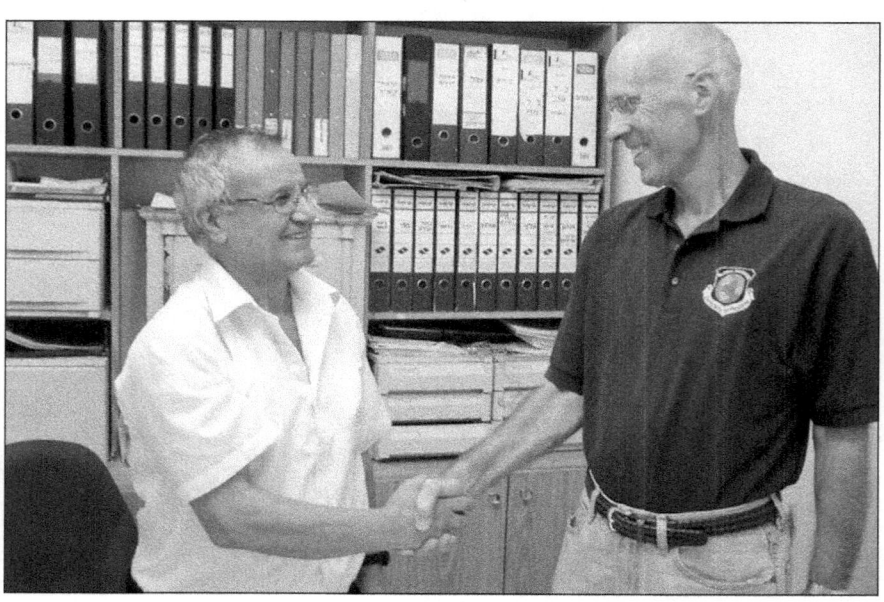

Ron with the Accountant. The final testimony of the goodness of God is how the accountant was willing to work with me, a foreigner, as I made payments in the several months that followed.

> **Friday, November 12**
>
> I rested and sent e-mail thank you notes and an outline of *The Malaria Survivor* (the original working title) to friends.

Pastor Ron and Char,

We received news of Ron's illness on Sunday evening, October 31. That morning before receiving the news, God had already laid on my heart regarding His healing (power). I had peace and confidence that God will perform mighty work and His name will be glorified.

This is what I shared with Sandy, Kevin, and his wife: In Pastor Ron's situation, we know God is going to do mighty things. Whether or not God heals Pastor Ron's body, Jesus Christ's name will be lifted up and be glorified. The "new" Pastor Ron, like the "resurrected Lazarus," will be a living testimony for God.

Sandy suggested that we fast and pray on Monday. Our prayers were to thank and praise God that He had already healed Pastor Ron … God will be glorified. Many will be drawn to Him and know Him and believe in Him.

Thank you for serving Him so faithfully … and for being a living testimony for our Lord Jesus Christ. May God strengthen you both physically and spiritually. You are always in our prayer.

Love in Christ,
Clayton

I am so happy to hear you are recovering well. I am very interested in hearing and reading about your experiences. I was discussing with Esther, "Guess who got malaria, ARDS, intubation, sedation, extubation, and as he recovers will recount his experiences by writing a book … that's right, Pastor Ron." You are a blessing to us. Praise God for His sovereign grace.

Kenny

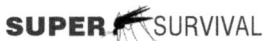

A very dear former colleague from South Korea, the president of Asia LIFE University wrote:

> Dr. Meyers:
>
> I am so glad to hear from you. Now you are still alive. When I heard from Char that you were in ICU and of her planning to ask Danny to come to Israel, I realized you were seriously ill. So I sent that message to headquarters and asked the secretary to send this message to all to pray for Dr. Meyers immediately. I received phone calls from many pastors. Praise the Lord. He saved your life. He healed you now. Yesterday, when the leaders met, I shared news of your health with them.
>
> Dr. Meyers, be strong and be healthy.
> Dr. Yeol Soom Eim

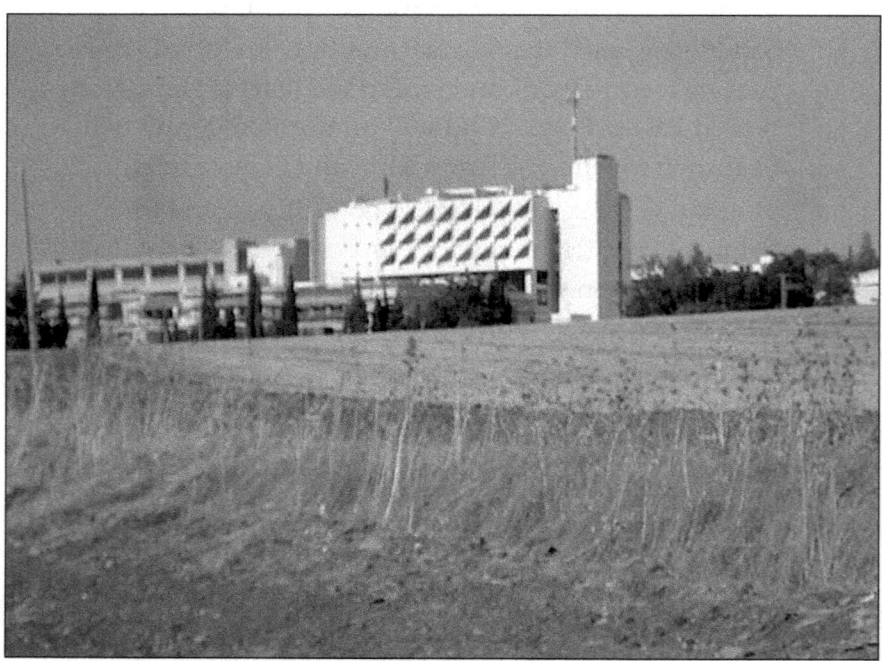

Poriya Hospital at a Distance. Every time we drive by the hospital, I recall the drama of those twelve days. I am more aware than ever before that God has a purpose for me in the years ahead.

> **Saturday, November 13**
>
> Char and I worshiped with a group of believers, rested, and sent more thank you e-mails and the outline of *The Malaria Survivor* to friends.

Dearest Professor Ron and Char,

I must first acknowledge God's faithfulness over your lives. This is a very touching but inspiring testimony of God's intervention and help. Thank God for answers to prayers, you are always in our mind ... I am waiting eagerly for the e-book.

Sincere and warm regards from the brethren,
Mark, Lausanne Younger Leaders Facilitator for Nigeria

This has been a time of renewal and healing for many as we examined our own dedication and prayer time with Him. The art of fasting came back into play ... This book sounds like a #1 for, after all, you had a world of people behind the scenes calling out to God in your behalf.

Rest and recuperate, my friend, because the race will pick up tempo once you say, "I'm ready and good to go."

Blessings,
Charlene

The healing you experienced taught us who were praying some valuable lessons about faith, the power of God to still perform miracles, and what happens when people join together to pray.

Aimee

> **Sunday, November 14**
>
> I began to write *The Malaria Survivor, Lessons for Life Learned Near Death*. The name was subsequently changed to *Super-Survival*.

> Dear Pastor,
>
> Thank God for healing your body.
>
> I have been blessed by your ministry in Cameroon through the internet lessons that you gave freely. I believe that you have contributed much for that which is eternal.
>
> May the Lord heal you speedily. 3 John 2.
>
> I am seriously considering my place in the world as a preacher and teacher of the Word and seeking divine guidance. There is unrest within me as I considered what is eternal to be more weighty than all temporary benefits in the world.
>
> Ndonwi

The above testimony is a sample of the reasons why Char and I are in this work — equipping and empowering people for leadership.

Thank you for continuing to join us in prayer and praise for our on-going strength and ministry.

AFTERWORD

Super-Survival is a word I made up, but you have probably already guessed its meaning. It means *beyond survival, more than survival, moving beyond mere recovery to becoming a better person than we were before the crisis.*

My friend, I was walloped with an extreme sickness. I almost went home to be with the Lord. Char almost became a widow. My life's work was almost cut off, to remain incomplete forever. As I lay physically beaten up, taken down, and hammered by thousands of malaria bacteria, my body almost succumbed to a mighty pestilence.

The key word here is *almost*. Those things almost happened, but they didn't.

Inside that broken, wounded, and battered body was a spirit fully focused on God. I communicated with God most of those hours. Not only did I come through, I experienced improvement, refinement, training, and softening. I learned how to pray, listen, and learn at a new depth.

The observations I share in these chapters cost a pretty price. I am sorry it takes such hardship to learn what I learned, but I am not willing to walk away without learning something valuable. I would not want to pay that price and come away from the trial only to remain the same. I will strive to become better for it. I claim improvement and so can you. I must. You must.

God's purpose for the hardships we experience is our personal

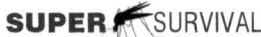

character development. Moving beyond mere recovery to developing godly moral fiber is far more important than regaining physical strength. In the eternal scope of things — in God's eyes — genuine moral fortitude is the quality God seeks to develop in us. This is how we can become real superheroes.

Each of the nine chapters has focused on one major lesson God taught me toward becoming a super-survivor. My reflections on these lessons along with my sickness and time in the hospital have convinced me that each of us has opportunities to become a super-survivor. We have the ability and potential not only to survive, but to thrive and become an enriched person. Why not strive for greatness and be all you can be?

> "Why not strive for greatness and be all you can be? God does not bring us through His training program for our development just barely, but rather triumphantly."

God does not bring us through His training program for our development just barely, but rather triumphantly. We can grow, learn, and be enriched because of it. Satan may mean the difficulty for harm, but God will use it for good if we let Him.

Reversals will occur. You too have and will experience difficult and even impossible situations. Yet we must learn how to hang on to God and use the situation to our advantage rather than let the enemy toss us around and rough us up at will. Through faith, confidence, prayer, and a teachable spirit, we will do more than just survive.

I write about what I learned from my twelve-day experience in the Poriya Hospital with the hope that you too will become a super-survivor. I want to learn these lessons more perfectly. If we learn how to learn, we can experience super-survival. We can and must learn from observation and experience.

The person who has learned how to learn from experience will ask,

"What do I learn from this?" instead of complaining, "Why did this happen to me?" He or she can continue to learn, grow, develop, and become a better person every year. The idea of learning from observation and experience is more fully developed in the first two chapters of *Habits of Highly Effective Christians* that I wrote some years ago.

May God grant to you the grace to experience this repeatedly each time you meet a reversal. God bless you, my fellow super-survivor. Let's move forward together.

You might like to know how I am doing now, physically, and how God has used the postponement of our ministry in Rwanda for His greater glory.

First, I want to thank God for all our precious friends who helped to sustain us through prayer during our dark trial while in the hospital, and even since. In many cases, I have been able to personally thank those who prayed with us through our dark valley. In other cases, I hope friends will receive my heartfelt expression here in print.

Physically, I continue to advance in my recovery. I am increasing the regimen to running an hour every two days and doing my weight-lifting routine with free weights on days I don't run. I don't run as fast as I used to because the sickness evidently affected my lungs. And even though I take less heart medication than when I was first released from the hospital, I am still on low doses of sedatives to quiet my heart. But I can run hard; and when I find mountains near wherever I travel, I remain challenged by them.

This is now two and a half years after my experience in Poriya Hospital. Just a year after my sickness, Char and I completed two months presenting eight different conferences, a special series, and a convention in Rwanda . We were well received. We know God has a plan for our continued fruitfulness since He spared my life. Our travel and conference schedule is continuing and now includes India and Russia. We call the conferences Leadership Empowerment

Conferences now. Though still active in Africa, we also travel to Europe and Asia, not just Africa.

Yours for Super-Survival!
Ron Meyers
Tiberius, Israel
July 2013

About the Author
Ron Meyers

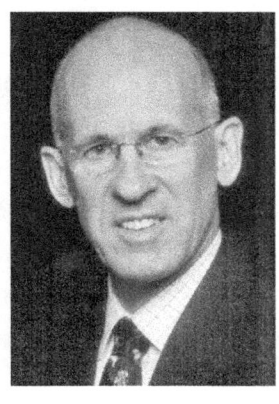

Ron Meyers was born in 1944 and raised in a pioneer pastor's home. In July 1965, he began pastoral ministry as a student pastor in a rural community seventy miles from the Bible College he attended in mid-Ohio.

From 1996 until 2006, he served as the Professor of Missions and Coordinator of the Master of Arts in Missions program in the School of Theology and Missions of Oral Roberts University. During those years, Ron traveled to African, Asian, European, and Middle Eastern nations during his summer breaks from university responsibilities.

He, with his wife, Char, have served more years outside the United States as pastors in Canada and missionaries in Korea, China, and Africa than their years in the U.S. Since January 2007, Ron and Char have lived in Africa, then Israel, and have traveled full-time to African, European, and Asian nations conducting Leadership Empowerment Conferences. Ron has a PhD in Intercultural Studies and Char has an EdD. The Meyers have two adult sons, one daughter-in-law, and eight grandchildren.

ABOUT THE AUTHOR

TOOLS FOR LEADERS

Leadership Empowerment Resources Website

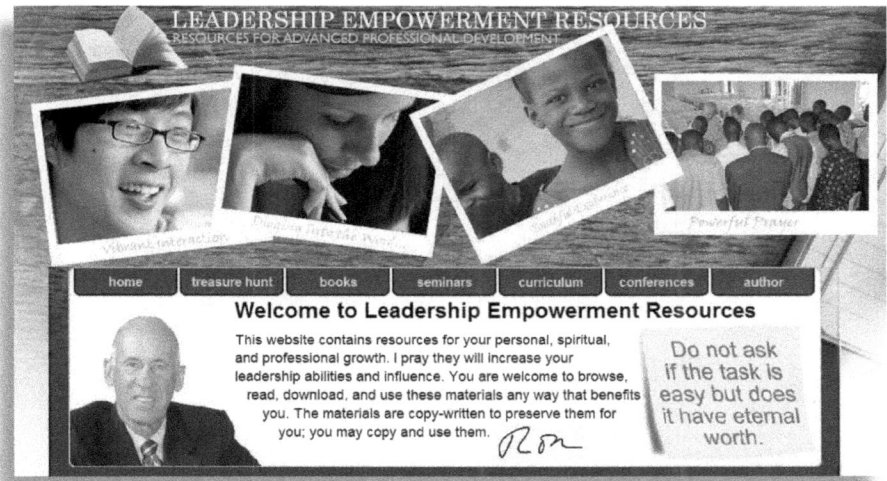

This website provides additional resources for Dr. Meyer's mission work abroad. It includes information on:

- **Books:** Resources written by Ron Meyers for expanding your wisdom and knowledge to use in any way that serves your purpose in helping to enrich the lives of Christians you know
- **Leadership Empowerment Conferences:** Ron and Char Meyers' Africa-based vehicle for strengthening His Church by training the leaders of churches
- **Treasure Hunt:** A Christian conversational game intended to be a catalyst for drawing out practical wisdom and understanding — treasures — from the hearts of Christians who enjoy wholesome conversational fun.

www.LEResources.com

Visit the Website

To read the code, download the QR Reader app for your cell phone and scan it.

OTHER BOOKS BY RON MEYERS

Habits of Highly Effective Christians Book and Study Guide

***Habits of Highly Effective Christians* Makes a Great Bible Study Program**

When Ron Meyers followed his passion for international missions work forty years ago, he never imagined the rich educational curriculum God had in store for him. A lifetime of spiritual challenges groomed him for his role at the School of Theology and Missions at Oral Roberts University in Tulsa, Oklahoma. Then, after ten years educating Christian ministry candidates at ORU and serving as Coordinator of the Master of Arts in Missions program, he and his wife moved to Africa where they now train pastors and missionaries throughout the southern African nations.

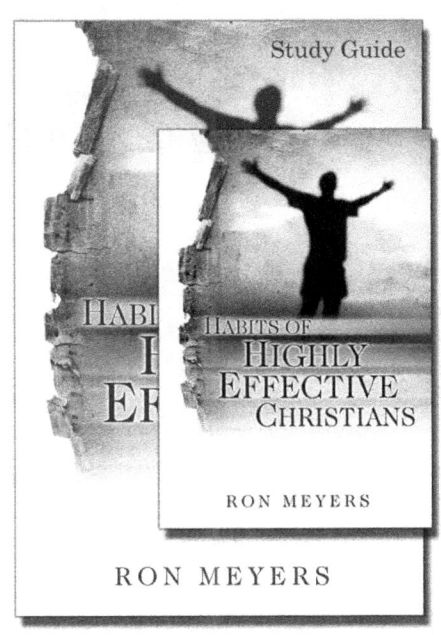

Meyers wrote his book with life application in mind. He weaves his stories into each habit by providing real-life, insightful, and applicable examples. *Habits of Highly Effective Christians* guides you through biblical resources for creating a rich tapestry with the fibers of your own life.

A Great Tool for Growth and Discussion

Proven to create rich discussions, *Habits of Highly Effective Christians* is perfect for small-group Bible studies or college classroom discussions. Meyers has also written the *Habits of Highly Effective Christians Study Guide*. Together, this study combo will etch biblical principles on every aspect of the lives you encounter.

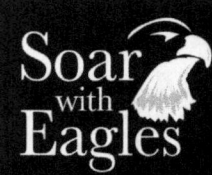

Books and e-books by Ron Meyers are available at online bookstores.

Quantity discounts are available by contacting Soar with Eagles (www.soarhigher.com).

OTHER BOOKS BY RON MEYERS

Rise to Seek Him:
The Joy of Effective Prayer

Allow God to Do Immeasurably More in Your Life

Effective prayer is more about becoming useful tools in God's hands than imposing our plans and desires on Him. In *Rise to Seek Him*, we learn that we accomplish much more when God uses us through prayer than when we try to use God to accomplish our objectives.

This is not just another book on prayer. Ron Meyers invites you to experiment for yourself how God can accomplish "immeasurably more" than you could ever ask or imagine. This book reveals fresh insights about the meaning of prayer — insights that were in the Bible all the time.

Rise to Seek Him offers practical solutions to the questions we all ask:

- How do we discipline ourselves to pray?
- How can we know what to pray for?
- Why is it difficult to pray?
- What is the focus of prayer?
- Does prayer really "work?"

This book testifies to the expansion in influence, effectiveness, and success possible with increased personal prayer.

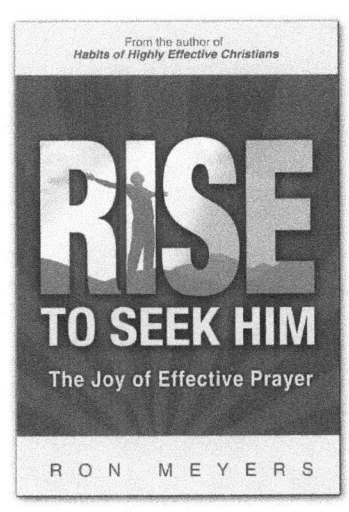

As in *Habits of Highly Effective Christians,* Meyers again describes self-discipline as a fruit of the Spirit to increase personal spiritual growth and improvement in public ministry. God-fearing Christians of any vocation who are serious about serving God at maximum levels of effectiveness will benefit from this book.

OTHER BOOKS BY RON MEYERS

Choose Your Character: 25 Bible Personalities Who Inspire Integrity

Powerful Lessons in Integrity

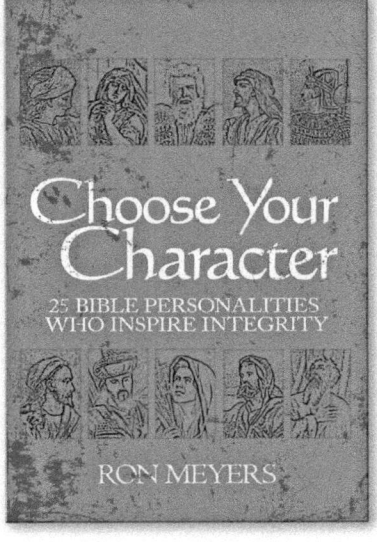

The writers of the Bible speak to us with their words, and the Bible's characters speak to us with their lives. Their powerful examples reveal the spiritual inspiration and brilliant insight the human writers and the divine Writer intended. Times, cultures, traditions, and societal values may change from century to century, but human nature does not.

We value people whose words and actions reflect their true thoughts and intentions. People of integrity purposely integrate their own thoughts, words, and behaviors. They work at making their own hearts and minds, thoughts and ideas consistent with the godly character portrayed in Scripture.

These twenty-five Bible personalities in *Choose Your Character* cultivate a desire to deepen the commitment to live a life of unfailing integrity. Their examples teach us how to increase our personal satisfaction and effectiveness while strengthening our ability to influence others.

OTHER BOOKS BY RON MEYERS

A Thoughtful Gift

Order *Super-Survival*
as a gift for family members and friends.

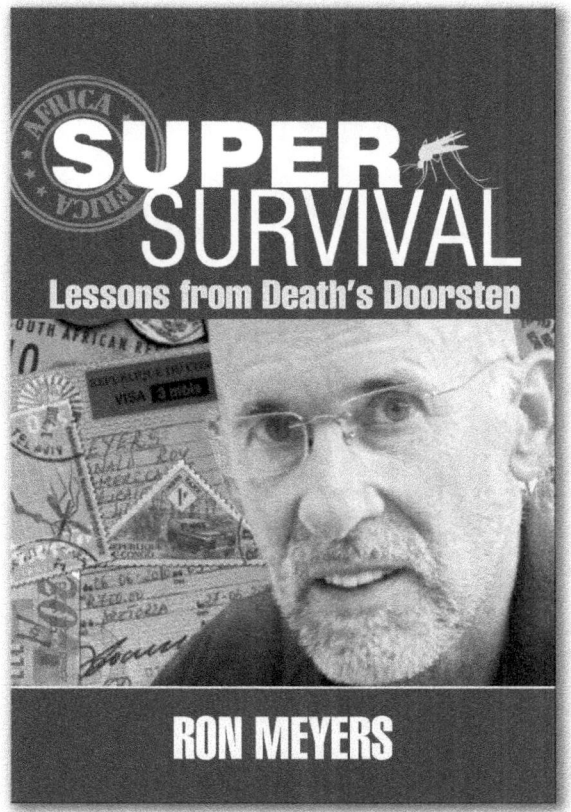

You can order additional copies at
online bookstores.

Quantity discounts are available by contacting
Soar with Eagles (www.soarhigher.com).

www.ingramcontent.com/pod-product-compliance
Lightning Source LLC
Chambersburg PA
CBHW070616050426
42450CB00011B/3071